Patrick

Tales from A Male Nurse

Patrick K S Poon

First published in Great Britain in 2013 by

Patrick K S Poon

www.pkspoon.co.uk

This book is dedicated to Shauna Jane O'Keeffe,

Our Granddaughter.

Acknowledgements

Special thanks for the help and editing from Bob Quinney. Thanks to Lindsey Faulkner for the design of the book front and back cover and Ryan, my eldest son for the technical help.

Thanks and support and ideas from Jane, my wife, children-- Ryan, Katherine, Thomas and Andy and Evan O'Keeffe.

Thanks for ideas and advice and support from Fraser and Lida Wight, Greg Heath , Peter White, Dan Liddicott, Jon Jacobs, Gabriel IP, Michael and Angela Lee, Natalie Greening and Victoria Melbourne. And the help from Helen Kirby, St. Dominic and Joy Robinson at BBC radio Cornwall and the help from Kam W C, Hong Kong.

To the tennis friends on Saturday mornings—Alistair Crooks, Bob Quinney, Malcolm Worth, Peter Innocent and Andrew Lea, Ashby Castle tennis club, Ashby-de-la-Zouch. Leicestershire.

Foreword

Every nurse has a tale to tell about his or her nursing life and I, a male nurse, have many tales. I am a keen tennis player and have been playing for more than twenty years at Ashby Castle Lawn Tennis Club, Ashby-de-la-Zouch. We played on Saturday mornings and, after tennis, went to the club house for coffee where we gossiped and resolved the crises of the world. I was an operational manager in the surgical unit at a nearby hospital and often used to tell the lads a nursing tale. They found the tales interesting, sometimes amusing, and said jokingly that I should write a book. I thought little of it at the time and eventually moved to Cornwall, semi-retired, to be nearer to the sea.

Two events triggered off my writing. The TV series, "Call the Midwife" glued me and my wife, a dedicated midwife and avid reader, to the screen, and one day, noticing Jennifer Worth's paperback "Call the Midwife" on the bedside table, I started reading it. Jennifer had once heard a conference speaker comment on the fact that no midwife had ever written a book about the process and drama of giving birth and as a result, she started writing. I did a Google search and found that no books had been written in the UK by a male nurse in general nursing, perhaps because there aren't many of us around.

FOREWORD

Last summer my daughter became ill but thank goodness she has now recovered. My wife went to Burton-on-Trent to help her for ten weeks, hardly coming home at all, and I found myself stranded in the village of St. Dominick in rural Cornwall. I live in an old cottage in a narrow lane with no street lights and high banks on either side. Through my windows I can see the rugged granite tors of Dartmoor and life is very still. It was in this tranquil environment, and occasionally in my son's house overlooking majestic Fistral bay, that I wrote my tales. The stories flowed from my mind as if the events had happened only weeks ago, some vivid and some so haunting. I enjoyed the journey back into the past.

All the names used in the book are fictitious. And any errors found are my faults.

This book is for Shauna, my granddaughter, to read when she is older, and for my four children who are unaware of the events I describe. It has been a mixture of relief, pleasure, and a little pain to commit my memories to print. It all happened so long ago -and I have never in my life written so many words.

Patrick K S Poon.
November, 2012.

Contents

Tale 1
Being a Male Nurse

'There is no escape for the odd one out.......'

Introduction.

I left Hong Kong on 9th April 1969, heading for Newmarket, England, to commence training as a pupil nurse. I was almost 19 years old and it was the first time I had left Hong Kong. My old college friend, Chanie, had arranged to meet me at Liverpool Street station, London, and travel with me to Newmarket. Chanie was a girl from our college in Hong Kong and we had known each other since we were fourteen years old. She had started training at Newmarket General Hospital a year before I arrived. She was a devout Christian and, unlike me, she always wanted to be a nurse.

My journey from Hong Kong had been tiring and complicated. There were two stops in the journey, the aeroplane broke down in Dubai and we were held up there for eighteen hours. Chanie, being a true friend, had requested a day off so that she could meet me in London but when I failed to arrive she returned to Newmarket wondering what had become of me.

I arrived at Heathrow airport very late and I then had to wait a long time for a coach to Liverpool Street station where I arrived some 20 hours behind schedule. My family was not well-off and I had worked in a mental hospital for nine months to save up the money for my flight. I also borrowed $500 (£35) from my brother to cover any emergencies that might arise.

I carried two heavy suitcases to the train and resumed my journey. I knew I had to make my way to Newmarket and wasn't afraid even though without Chanie to act as a guide I wasn't quite sure where the town was. The train seemed to take hours to get to Cambridge, the nearest stop to Newmarket, and it was dark, cold and raining when I arrived. Standing on the deserted platform I felt all alone in the world, hungry, tired and lost. It seemed a long way from Hong Kong.

There were no buses so I had to spend £15, a fortune in 1969, to hire a taxi from Cambridge to Newmarket General Hospital, some thirteen miles away. It was raining heavily when I arrived and to Sister Parr, who happened to be standing in the doorway as I walked towards the entrance; I must have looked like a drowned cat. I didn't know at the time that she was to become my clinical tutor. Months later she told me that when she first saw me she felt so sorry for me, a young lad from a busy city in another continent starting a new life in the quiet market town of Newmarket in rural England.

I came into the world of nursing quite by accident. My father's brother was an orderly in the war but people called him a semi-doctor in old China, as he helped doctors to care for the sick during the war. My parents didn't discourage me to go into nursing. I knew I didn't want an office job. I was no good with a hammer and screw drivers and I was not good at mathematics either, so I tried nursing. I quite liked it and I have stayed in the profession ever since. When I entered the profession I didn't know much about anything, let alone male nurses in the largely female world of nursing.

****

Forty years ago women dominated the workforce by a ratio of about ten to one although in psychiatric nursing the ratio was reversed. Beginning my career in general nursing I was very conscious of being a member of a minority group and at times felt like the odd one out.

In those days nurses were poorly paid, hence many trained male nurses would apply for more senior positions in order to earn more money, often necessitating moving to another hospital. Female nurses, after training, tended to stay at a hospital longer because their husbands often had a job there and they found it more difficult to move. The promotion of men rather than women had made many women resentful because most of their bosses were men younger than themselves.

Junior, less experienced nurses were paid less than those with more experience and we accepted that, therefore men, especially married men, felt they needed to earn more money to support a family; hence they were more willing to move farther away to secure a better job.

However, on the wards, especially in the sixties and the seventies, many of the ward sisters were single and seemed to favour the male nurses. Perhaps it was because they lacked male company but whatever it was we often felt we were the blue eye staff on the ward. Certainly, during my allocations as a trainee nurse, the vast majority of the ward sisters liked me. It might have been that I was a good worker, willing to learn and that I got on well with the female nurses. Many other female nurses seemed to like working with male nurses too. They said that we were more straight forward and less "bitchy" to work with than their female colleagues.

There were, obviously, many instances where male nurses "chatted up" female trained staff or student nurses while some male nurses found themselves doing some of the worst jobs on the ward.

In the world of nursing, because of the imbalance between the sexes, male nurses found they had a large pool of women from which to choose to ask out. Some courted them and married them and many marriages worked very well as both partner understood what each other's job was all about. When I became a staff nurse and later on a charge nurse, I was always aware of the fact that, in meetings, the overwhelming majority of the people attending were women. In spite of the obvious attractions of being surrounded by colleagues of the opposite sex, a hospital could be quite a lonely place to live. Some male nurses preferred to keep themselves to themselves and found it difficult to mix with others. They were a lonely breed and felt alone in a people-centred job.

Doctors sometimes seemed to think men could get away with things on the ward that female nurses couldn't get away with. It's true that female nurses did become envious of at times because we were allocated jobs that were perceived to be easier or more prestigious, and we were chosen to help with doctors more frequently. In those days doctors were mostly male and I knew of a few ward sisters who preferred to work with male rather than female nurses.

More male than female nurses, including staff nurses and charges nurses, could be found working in operating theatres, elderly care wards and colleges of nursing. Working as a charge nurse on an acute medical ward and surgical ward was quite a rare breed. Some ward sisters asked me why I preferred working on such busy wards and my answer would be that I was young and wanted to learn the knowledge and skills required of acute nursing, which would help me to progress in the future. Some years later I worked in a hospital in a deprived region and we had to deal with diseases such as scabies and tuberculosis, conditions often caused by poverty and deprivation. I acquired skills and knowledge which I was able to put to good use in later years when I moved on to education.

Working as a male ward sister in charge of predominately female staff could be challenging. When I first became a charge nurse, I felt uneasy as I could sense an air of envy from some female staff nurses, especially the younger ones. Perhaps it was because I was Chinese or male, I wasn't sure. They observed the way I spoke and the way I wrote reports. I had to be cautious but it was to my advantage that the middle-aged senior sister on the ward had an abrupt manner whereas I was much younger, more dynamic and had better social skills. I was more interested in teaching and the senior ward sisters almost invariably asked me to teach the student nurses, which I enjoyed.

The local college liked me because I was more interested in teaching than the senior sister and I was very pleased when a report I had written about a student was used as an example by the senior tutor of the local College of Nursing. I had commented on the unprofessional conduct of student on my ward and used an example of her whistling during ward duties. From then on, the local College of Nursing frequently asked for examples from my reports.

Having worked for five years as a charge nurse, I was promoted to nursing officer of the surgical unit. The previous nursing officer retired and I was asked to replace him on a temporary basis. Sometime later I was asked to apply for the post and was offered the job on a permanent basis.

All the ward sisters under me then were younger and female and it was a strange feeling to be in charge of them because they were more experienced in their own specialities which included ear, nose and throat and gynaecology. However, the surgical unit ran very smoothly.

There were sensitive areas outside the practise of nursing. For instance, I had to consult ward sisters for their opinion on uniforms and nurses' caps. No men would dare to interfere on such topics as these.

But times have changed. There were procedures and routine on the ward that happened in the olden days that were not happening now. For instance, part of the important care for patients on the wards was diet. Food trolleys were taken to the ward and it was an important role for the nurse in charge to arrange different types of diet of food for patients, such as weighing out correctly portions of carbohydrate food for diabetics. If we had leftovers, we might save some food for some junior doctors who were so busy, working for 18 hours without having opportunities to eat food. At times, I felt so sorry for them and offered them food kept from the trolley. These doctors were very grateful to be fed. These days have gone now. All food were now cooked and chilled some four weeks before, the so-called 'cook-chilled food' for all patients.

All food were plated and given to patients regimentally. Ice creams were not allowed to be kept in the fridge because of health and safety issues.

On reflection, nursing was very good for me and gave me a fair standard of living. My experiences in acute medical and surgical nursing gave me valuable medical knowledge. That might be the reason why, after I left the NHS, I had no difficulty in obtaining a post in a nursing home. Four years later, after leaving the NHS, I became a lecturer, teaching on and assessing NVQ courses. I felt that I was blessed by my thorough training and wide experience. I had become an advocate for nursing, even though in my earlier days I was frequently told off by my senior who used to tell me that in those days of uncertainty, many trained nurses were unable to find a job. I disagreed with her and said that if we did not become advocates for nursing, then nobody would, and that the country would always need nurses to look after the old, the sick and the disabled.

The subsequent chapters of this book are mostly true stories, based on personal experiences. Some of those experiences were sad, some happy and some rewarding. Writing it was a painstaking process. Some facts were almost forgotten but they came back to me, often in the middle of the night, as if the incident had happened only yesterday.

I hope that you will enjoy reading them.

Tale 2

Jason's Tragic Accident – 1968

'Compassion will cure more sins than condemnation.'

I was born and bred in Hong Kong. I was eighteen years old and was expected to pass my GCEs with flying colours because I was good at school and always in the top ten of a class of 40 students. But unfortunately I didn't do well at all. I passed only two subjects, namely Chinese and English history, and I was devastated.

My father offered to support me for another year in the same class but my family was poor and money was tight, so I declined his offer. In Hong Kong, we had to pay for college education so I did private tutoring in English for a group of children during the day and went to evening classes to study to retake my examinations the following year. Unfortunately, I didn't pass any more subjects.

I did not have a goal as to what to do with my life. I did know that I didn't want an office job because it would bore me. Since I was the youngest son I was quite protected and manual labour was not really an option. Using a screwdriver or hammer wasn't my strength and I once took a job as a telephone technician trainee and hated it. It was the only time I cried because I hated the job. My mother would console me and I resigned after a short time.

One of my good friends in the college was called Old Chan and she had wanted to be a nurse for many years. She influenced my decisions and helped me to find my path in life. My Father's brother was an untrained nurse in China. During the War, he had helped doctors' to care for the sick and my Father encouraged me to be a nurse. Hence, when I saw a suitable job advertised in the South China Morning Post I applied for it and commenced training as a pupil nursing auxiliary. It was not a post as student nurse and I could not become a trained nurse that way. However, it was a job, relatively well paid and it could give me good insight into the world of nursing.

The post involved working in mental nursing at a mental hospital on the outskirts of the city, in the New Territory. In 1968, the hospital was in a rural area and I had to take a bus to the location. From the bus stop, I walked for 10 minutes uphill, through the village to the hospital. At night, there were no streetlights and it was very quiet but things were very safe then and it did not trouble me to walk alone in the darkness.

Because of the journey and the shift duties in the evenings and early mornings, we had to live in the nurses' home. There were 10 of us in a group and I shared a room with Jason. The hospital was huge, with many wards and large grounds.

Jason was old-fashioned, quite small and had short hair. He was softly-spoken, sincere and seemed a nice guy. He had been in Hong Kong for three years since escaping from China. He was a strong swimmer and had escaped from China illegally by swimming to Hong Kong, spending some two or three hours in the water, with the help of a basketball. In our college days, it was not uncommon to see corpses floating in Hong Kong harbour, the unfortunate Chinese escapees who drowned before reaching safety. They had died trying to escape the harsh life in China under Chairman Mao.

Jason was 23 years old, quite a bit older than me, and I liked him. Like me, he wore glasses, but more frequently than I did. The induction course was three weeks long and gave us some insight into what to do on the ward. At weekends we went home to Hong Kong to enjoy our two days off. Months passed by quickly and Jason and I seldom met because we were working on different wards and often working different shifts, but we got on well together.

The work was quite boring because most routine duties were done by the less seriously ill patients and the orderlies would look after those less able to care for themselves. The orderlies were big chaps which was often useful when handling troublesome or violent mental patients. A high proportion of the staff had been there for many years, most of the patients for more than 20 years and were unlikely ever to be discharged. Most patients seemed to be suffering from severe neurosis and psychosis. I was told that they were the outcasts of society and would not fit into the social environment outside. I was advised not to feel sorry for them as they were unaware of the nature of their illness. We were advised to stand with our backs to the wire fence so that we could not be attacked from behind. My role seemed to be helping the trained nurses to give out drugs twice to three times a day. That was the part of the work that I liked best, the knowledge of the drugs.

Six months into the job, Jason and I were working on the

same ward, a ward for schizophrenic patients, one of three wards in the same category. One day I reported for duty on the late shift. The atmosphere in the ward didn't seem quite right, as if something serious had happened. I inquired and was told that Jason had been hit on the face by a psychotic patient and broken glass from his spectacles had gone into his eyes. Jason's eyes were badly injured and he was taken to hospital for an emergency operation. Some of the ward staff felt anxious and unsettled. As I was sharing a room with Jason, I was asked by the charge nurse if I would like to visit him in hospital. I readily agreed and was taken to see him.

The patient who hit him was a very quiet man in his thirties, always muttering to himself on the ward or in the yard. An accident report was written and it was noted that incidents like this, especially involving attacks on staff, were very rare. The charge nurse had little to say but seemed to be annoyed.

Jason's relatives had already visited him in hospital and gone home to bring him some clothes. He had already had the operation and was fully awake.

"It's Patrick, Jason" I said as I approached the bed.

"Hello Patrick," he said in a calm voice.

"Sorry to see you like this." I was a bit choked, seeing half of his face was bandaged.

"Not to worry, they told me that some pieces of glass were removed from my eyes and I shall be ok."

"Thanks God," I said, taking his hand." Is there anything I can get for you?'

"No, it's ok, not to worry, I'm young and I shall be fine."

"Really?" I had led quite a sheltered life and felt very sorry and sad for Jason, but pleased that he seemed to be accepting the accident so well. Much better than I was in fact.

"In China, there were far more and worse tragedies than mine," Jason remarked.

"I admire your courage. Thank goodness things are going to be ok."

"The patient must have been hallucinating and just hit me," said Jason.

"Bugger him!" I said angrily.

"Don't be angry, that's life." Jason was calm and forgiving.

To me, it was the most real and close encounter with tragedy I had seen. The fact that it had happened to someone I knew, my roommate, disturbed me more than it had him.

I stayed with him for 45 minutes, promised him that I would visit him again and then the transport took me back to the mental hospital.

The following afternoon, I was on a late shift again. At the reporting or handing over, there was a tense atmosphere on the ward, as if someone had died. The report was sharp and swift and I followed all the staff through the back door.

Nearly all the staff had gathered in a room at the back of the building, near the patient's dormitory and I sensed something was going on. I was relatively new and just waited. The charge nurse was there and the patient who had hit Jason was led into the room, muttering to himself. The charge nurse, without hesitation, punched the patient in the stomach. The patient fell backwards and the big orderlies started to join in, beating the patient quite severely with their clenched fists. Other staff joined in and I felt that I too had to join them. I kicked him three or four times but couldn't hit him any more as the victim was black and blue, totally defenceless and delirious. He was lying there motionless, quiet and subdued. Later on I discovered that this was a ritual procedure in the hospital whenever accidents like this occurred.

The patient had no relatives and it was reported the following day that he was unable to attend occupational therapy as he had fallen down in the bathroom the previous night.

The next day was my day off and I went home. My mother rubbed my foot with healing oil as it was badly bruised as a result kicking the patient. My parents were not surprised by the incident as they knew that worse things happened in mental hospitals, but the incident made me think hard about whether I should continue working in psychiatric hospitals. Some time later I checked on the patient because I felt guilty about hitting him. He wasn't looking badly injured, considering what he had been through, and he was able to eat and drink fairly normally.

From my nine months of working there, I found that I liked many aspects of nursing generally, but I wasn't so keen on mental nursing. Sometime later I applied and was successful in obtaining a place in nurse training in England.

Jason recovered well from his operation and after 3 months he returned to work. He stayed in mental nursing for many years. The patient also recovered well and stayed in the hospital for his remaining years. Jason didn't keep in contact and I often wondered which of us this episode in his life had affected most. He seemed at the time to have taken it so well.

I heard later that Jason had left the hospital and went to Sydney, Australia, for further training and had become a trained psychiatric nurse. An old friend told me recently that Jason was still living in Sydney and was married now with two children.

Tale 3
Johnny and One for the Road

'That I might drink and leave the world unseen ...' John Keats.

I started training as a pupil nurse in Newmarket General Hospital in 1969. It was a small hospital in a quiet market town in East Anglia, but famous for being one of the horse-racing capitals of the world. The matron had accepted my written application from Hong Kong, but today an applicant would be required to attend an interview. I had made forty or more applications to various hospitals in Britain and received two positive replies. My successful application enabled me to obtain a visa and passport to come to England for training. The hospital no longer exists and the building is now a nursing home.

At the beginning I felt that most of my roles were domestic. I laid the tables, collected the used cutlery and dishes afterwards, and helped to feed the helpless patients three times a day, breakfast, lunch and dinner. I washed and cared for weak and frail patients as well, but I was never asked to do the washing up. That was a role performed by the domestics. Some years before my arrival, coal fires had to be made to keep the ward warm, but by the time I commenced my training we had central heating. I found it rewarding to help the sick, but if you look around any hospital ward today you will find these mundane, essential tasks being carried out by care assistants. I think today's students are missing a valuable opportunity to develop early on the essential personal, social and caring skills, that we learnt in our early years.

We had to work shifts and if we were lucky we might have one weekend off in four. It was necessary to work early or late shifts and most of the time, split shifts, which weren't very popular amongst the trainees. A split shift involved working from seven thirty in the morning until two o'clock in the afternoon and then from five in the afternoon until eight at night. Today it is seldom anyone has to work split shifts.

One late shift I went on duty on an acute medical ward and was asked to "special" a patient. There were no intensive care units in those days and very few side rooms. To "special" meant that it was my sole responsibility to care for that patient during my shift. He was called Johnny, a nineteen year old truck driver with a serious heart problem, unusual in one so young. He was so breathless that he collapsed as he was driving through Newmarket, while en route from Yorkshire to Felixstowe. I introduced myself and greeted him.

"How are you feeling today?"

"Pretty rough," Johnny replied in a strong northern accent. He was breathing oxygen from a 100% venti mask attached to a cylinder, and being hydrated by intravenous infusion. He was thin, pale and his eyes were dark-rimmed and sunken.

"Sorry to hear that," I said, "I'm your nurse and I'll be with you during this shift. Just call me or press the bell if you need anything, ok?' He read my name badge as I spoke.

"Thanks," he said gratefully.

"Would you like a drink?"

"Yes please." His lips were dry and I took a beaker, held up his head and sat him up to help him with his drink of Lucozade, for which he expressed his appreciation.

"Oh, I feel really ill!" Johnny whispered weakly.

I tried to reassure him. "Don't worry, and don't exert yourself, I'm here to help you."

In those days it was the norm in nursing and medical practice for any patient with a heart complaint or heart attack to have complete bed rest for five days, except perhaps to visit the toilet in a wheelchair. At mealtimes they would be fed by nurses whereas today, patients would have one day's bed rest and would be allowed to eat and drink freely without assistance. It was not easy for me to feed a young man of a similar age to me, especially as he was so poorly and I took my time to feed him, spoonful by spoonful.

"I hear you drive for a living?" I asked, trying to engage him in small talk.

"Yes, and brick laying," Johnny replied, "It's quite unusual to be a male nurse, isn't it?'

"Yes, I suppose it is. I am hoping to be a trained nurse."

"Good for you. I wish I had more skills."

"You are young enough to change and learn more skills," I said encouragingly.

"Thanks, but at the moment I feel so ill and weak."

"Have any other members of your family had any problems of this kind?" I asked

"No. They say that this happened because I was paid too much!"

"I'm not sure what you mean," I said, anxious to know more.

"Well, I guess I'm paid four or five times as much as you, so making and spending money is easy for me."

"Oh?" I remarked, quite taken aback.

"Yes, and because it was so easy I became involved with a gregarious, hard drinking crowd and started to drink a lot?'

"How much do you drink?" I asked

"I suppose I've been drinking about twenty pints a day for the past years."

"Really," I tried to conceal how shocked I was. "Didn't anyone advise you how dangerous that could be?"

"No one at all," he replied. "I'm not close to my family."

"I understand the hospital has contacted your family."

"But they won't come," he said, showing no emotion, "they have no transport and live so far away."

"I am sorry," I sympathised. I was given the impression he didn't come from a close and caring family.

After a few days Johnny was feeling a little better although he found getting out of bed a bit of a struggle. The doctors were baffled as to why a young man had such an enlarged heart, apparently caused by excessive alcohol consumption. His relatives didn't come to see him and although he had plenty of cash in his pockets, he was viewed as quite a sad, lonely young figure, on a ward where nearly all the patients were from nearby villages. He wasn't very well educated and, drinking apart, seemed to have led a sheltered life.

One day, I was trying to reassure him because he was feeling sorry for himself and was wondering what the future would hold for him. "I wish somebody had told me that too much drinking could harm me" he remarked sadly.

I didn't know what to say to him except to continue to encourage him, remind him that he was young and that would get better soon.

Two days later, in the early hours of the morning, Johnny had a cardiac arrest and the doctors were unable to save him.

I remained in hospital nursing for another 27 years but I have never since seen another young death like this from heart troubles. Poor Johnny was a unique and unusual patient.

1970

Tale 4
Catheters and Tennis – 1982

'For this relief much thanks ...' William Shakespeare, Hamlet

I was a charge nurse and male ward sister on a surgical ward for three years. It was an exciting, volatile ward in which we all worked hard, but the job was a very rewarding one. The turnover of patients in the ward was quick. Every day was different and it was less depressing than a medical ward, where I once had seven deaths over one weekend.

It was seven thirty in the evening and I was on duty on my ward, all part of the job of a shift worker. I was at my desk, writing the report for the shift, when I felt a friendly hand on my shoulder.

"Ah, there you are, Patrick."

"Oh, what's that?" I asked, looking round at a familiar face.

"Two pieces of best sirloin steak for you and your wife," the visitor replied.

"That's very kind of you, we'll enjoy that. How are you keeping?" I knew he had been a patient of mine and I was trying hard to remember his name.

"You can't remember my name, can you?" he said, looking a little disappointed.

"Sorry, squire, I know you were the retention of urine, at the corner of that bay."

"I can't blame you, must have hundreds of patients."

"We do, it's a fast turnover on this surgical ward."

"Denis, the name's Denis."

"Yes, of course. You're looking well Denis."

"Thanks to you, I feel well. Do you remember what you said to me?"

Denis was admitted to the surgical ward with an acute urine retention problem and had not passed urine for four days. His abdomen was almost up to his chin and he was in agony. He looked very pale, with a fast pulse and low blood pressure. He desperately wanted to urinate and could not, quite a common complaint on a surgical ward. The doctors were all very busy, either admitting new emergency patients, more seriously ill than Denis, or engaged in the operating theatre. Denis had been waited for two hours.

The telephone rang. "Charge nurse speaking," I answered.

"Hi, it's David." He was the surgical registrar, telephoning from the operating theatre.

"Hello David."

"Can you do me a favour, Patrick, all the doctors are busy? Could you put a catheter in the new patient? He hasn't peed for 4 days."

"Sure," I replied.

"Good, I knew you would, you've done it many times before and you taught my houseman how to do it. Is the patient a big man?

"Fairly large," I said.

"Better put in a big size then, ok."

"Fine, leave it with me."

"Thanks, Patrick."

Being a trained and experienced male nurse, I was frequently asked to catheterise male patients to help the busy doctors. I didn't mind as it was all part of the service and invariably a great relief to patients.

A nurse set up the trolley for me with a Foley catheter size 22 and helped me with the procedure. I washed my hands thoroughly and the nurse helped me put all the equipment that I needed on the sterile dressing pack. I swabbed the patient's groin area and applied an anaesthetic ointment, waiting a few minutes for it to take effect.

I said what I usually said jokingly to patients before this procedure, to put them at ease. "I'm going to put this catheter inside you. I might hurt you for minute but after that you will love me forever." I learnt this from an Australian doctor who worked with us for eighteen months. He used to say things in a rather crude but very effective way. Sometimes after an operation, he would say to elderly patients, "Pop, if you can piss against the wall in the toilet, you can go home because that means you have a good stream!"

The catheter went in quite smoothly without any of the obstruction I thought I might encounter. Denis was likely to have an enlarged prostate gland which was the usual cause of the retention of the urine. He took a deep breath as I inserted the catheter into his bladder but I clamped it after it had drained one and half litres into the urine bag.

'Denis, are you okay?'

"What a relief. You are a saint, Patrick. Thanks very much, you're a great chap."

"I hope I didn't hurt you too much."

"Not at all, I feel so much better already."

"We'll relieve you again in thirty minutes and every thirty minutes until it's drained off, ok? If we drain off too much too quickly you might go into shock."

"That's fine, Patrick."

Denis went on to have investigations that revealed an enlarged prostate, for which an operation was necessary. He asked me for advice and I told him that following the operation he must drink up to three or four litres a day, as it was essential for him to rinse the bladder otherwise he would be in clot retention afterwards. I said he could drink more or less anything, fruit juices, lager or water, the important thing was that he must drink. He asked me what the consequences were of not drinking and I told him that my neighbour went into hospital for the same operation but he was not in the habit of drinking much at all. He drank very little after his operation and within a short time he died.

"I didn't mean to frighten you, Denis. Drinking in order to rinse the bladder, or renal dialysis as we call it, is a very good habit to get into, provided you don't overdo the alcohol" I explained.

Denis had the operation, made a very good recovery and was discharged. We had many patients like Denis and the overwhelming majority made a complete recovery and went back home. Because we had so many patients admitted with retention of urine, I soon forgot him.

Years later, I went into education and taught carers how to catheterise patients. I was a keen tennis player and after a game, my mates and I used to talk about many things over a cup of coffee. We solved many a world crisis and sometimes, by way of a diversion, I entertained them with my catheter stories. I kept a dressing pack, including a supply of catheters, in the boot of my car, ready to teach carers how to perform the procedure and my tennis-playing friends used to tease me about it, saying that if players misbehaved on court, I would fetch my kit from the car and catheterise them!

Tale 5
Love and Lust on the Wards

'Is it, in Heav'n, a Crime to Love Too Well' Alexander Pope.

I was born in Hong Kong in 1949, the youngest son in a family of six children. We were raised by our mother, grandmother and father and I led a quiet, sheltered life. I was given no opportunity to cook or to use tools, not even a screwdriver, consequently I have never been any good at DIY.

In 1968 I became a pupil nurse auxiliary in a mental hospital, one of ten young men in the class. Most of us were eighteen years old but the oldest, William, was twenty-four. William was quite a mature man and had previously had several jobs, but for most of us, it was our first.

Our tutor was Sister Edith, only twenty-six, but with a successful career behind her. She was trained in Hong Kong, qualified as a staff nurse and was so good at her job that she was quickly promoted to ward sister. She was good looking, enthusiastic, energetic and very young to be a nurse tutor.

Edith was very good to us, down to earth and quite attached to our group. She had trained two groups previously and said our group was better and keener to learn. She was very friendly and gave me lifts from Kowloon to the New Territories, about an hour's drive from the hospital. She knew some songs that I knew and we would often sing them happily together. She liked to dress trendily, which, in the 1960s, usually meant short skirts or mini-dresses and she looked quite spectacular. I thought I was very lucky to have such a kind-hearted lady as a tutor and chauffeur.

She taught me a lot about nursing and because the group often had dinners and other gatherings together, my social skills also improved. We were intrigued to discover she was living with a married man, but when we got to know her better she told us that her heart had once been broken when a love affair had ended acrimoniously. Sometimes, at parties, we played machong and she could be seen playing footsie under the table with her married partner but we took no notice. I thought that we students were so junior to Edith in terms of status that perhaps we shouldn't be socialising with her, but she obviously enjoyed our company so we didn't complain.

Some of us left after nine months to be trained as nurses in England and Edith held a farewell party for us. A group of us, including William, went to Runwell mental hospital in Essex to train as psychiatric nurses and others to several different hospitals, but all of us who went to England stayed in contact. After six months or so we arranged a reunion in Essex and were quite surprised when William and Edith turned up, holding hands, obviously quite close, and looking very much like a couple. Apparently, Edith had come to England to do a nursing course in a London hospital but some of us thought that might have been an excuse to be with William. Some time later we discovered that they had been living together for many months.

Shortly after the reunion I learnt that after completing her nine months course Edith had returned to Hong Kong and she and William drifted apart. A few years later I heard that she had married and had a son but she never replied to my letters. Perhaps she was a little ashamed of her past and wanted to make a fresh start.

I often wondered why such an attractive woman had led such an unstable love life, but still I felt she was a very nice person and as time went on I concluded that she might have had personal problems to resolve, including issues relating to rejection, love and sex. On reflection, no other woman since has been so friendly, helpful and kind to me as Edith was when I was taking my first faltering steps in nursing. It is a kind of unconditional feeling that I treasure and I have never had cause to feel that way since.

As the years went by I tried to keep in contact and once, on a visit to Hong Kong, I enquired about her, but it was to no avail and I never met her again. Although I didn't know her for very long, Edith was certainly a helpful and influential figure in my early life.

My first hospital in Newmarket employed a large number foreign staff. Most of the cooks were Spanish - young, happy, carefree and very popular with the local staff. I was living in the male nurses' home, quite near to some of the Spanish cooks. A few of the women took a fancy to some of them and it was quite common to hear passionate sounds and the creaking of beds emanating from the cook's quarters. Advances were also made to some of the Chinese students.

In the small rural town of Newmarket, most of the women were, by modern standards, old fashioned and very respectable. I worked for four months with enrolled nurse

Helen who was always so kind to patients and staff. One Indian houseman, Rakesh, liked Helen very much and they often went out together. Rakesh was a gentleman, well-spoken, conservative and the staff thought he and Helen were well-suited.

They had been going out together for nearly a year and everything seemed to be progressing satisfactorily, when one day, Rakesh was found dead, hanging from a rope in an outbuilding at the back of the hospital. The news horrified the hospital staff but foul play was not suspected and it was subsequently established that he had committed suicide by hanging, the reason being the strong opposition from his family in India to his relationship with an English girl of a different faith and culture. We tried to console Helen but she was heartbroken, devastated and looked dreadful. Why hadn't the young doctor spoken to anyone about the problem before killing himself? We will never know, but we do know that he was deeply in love with an English woman and knew that his family would never accept her as his wife.

One night, my first time on night duty, I was thinking life seemed to be all work, sleep and eating. Fortunately, I slept well, often like a log, for eight hours during the day. It was the early seventies and staff was thin on the ground. Quite often we students were left in charge of a ward, although a night sister was in overall charge. Today, such a practice would never be allowed.

The night sister, Jeannette, was middle-aged, unmarried, slightly built and quite friendly. I must have appeared an innocent young man to her, and she often commented that I was naïve, but conscientious and willing to learn. I was in charge of seven patients on a children's ward, an easy job because they were so friendly and undemanding.

One night one of the children, a young girl, Rosemary, couldn't sleep and was feeling miserable. There was little to do in the ward and I tried to console her by holding her hands and speaking softly. She asked where I was from and I described what it was like to live in Hong Kong. She was missing her mother, but soon drifted off to sleep.

I was an inquisitive person, some would say nosey, and at times I was bored. When it was quiet I would sometimes look to see what was going on outside the ward. The long corridor was very quiet but well lit and one of the doors off the corridor opened onto the surgical ward. When I was sure Rosemary was asleep I wandered onto the corridor, peered through the glass panel in the door and saw the night sister, Jeannette, and a young nurse, Mary, apparently doing the rounds. As I looked they went into an alcove in the ward where they couldn't be seen by the patients and fell into each other's arms, kissing and cuddling like lovers. I hurried away, shocked, confused and a little disgusted at what I had witnessed.

The following morning, in the canteen, there was the usual gossip, banter and small-talk amongst the staff, most of whom had worked together for years and knew each other well, unlike the trainees who felt like passers-by. I just ate and listened.

"Night Sister Jeannette was on duty last night so everything will be in place this morning," I heard someone say.

"Yes, she's very efficient and easy to work with," said another.

"I like Sister Jeannette."

"Yes, so do I." They drank their coffee and smirked knowingly.

"Was Mary was on the surgical ward last night?'

"Yes, the two of them were together, as usual."

'Well, they are both very capable nurses, it's a free country and they can do what they like, so long as it's legal."

"Yes, I agree. Even in the quiet little town of Newmarket!'

They saw me smiling and one of them said, "You're new here, aren't you?"

"Yes, and I've been on nights only for a week."

'How do you like it?'

"Not bad at all, thanks."

"Good. Do they have many lesbians in Hong Kong?"

"I wouldn't know," I replied, feeling slightly embarrassed.

I had two nights off and then went back to night duty on the paediatric ward where the day sister was waiting for me to hand over the report.

After giving me the report, sister said to me, "Be careful not to get too attached to young patients here, Mr. Poon."

"Oh, why?'

'Do you remember Rosemary, the young girl at the corner of the childrens' ward?'

"Yes, she couldn't sleep a few nights ago night and I talked to her."

'Well, she didn't want to be discharged yesterday and she was talking about you all the time. She told her mum she was in love with you."

"Oh dear!" I was almost speechless.

"Never mind, children are like that, but be very careful in future."

I felt I was just being kind and helpful to the girl and treated her as a child, but she became almost obsessed with me.

It was a very unusual and unnerving experience and one from which I learnt a valuable lesson.

1969

Tale 6
Dr Tash and Mr Smilie

'Gold is tested by fire, man by Gold.' - Confucius.

1979 was my first year of working as a male ward sister. I was learning fast, enjoying the work and was aware that there were many good and conscientious doctors in the National Health Service. Some were very righteous people who would treat all patients the same, whatever their social standing or status in society and some would not undertake private medicine because they thought their NHS salaries were sufficiently generous to enable them to enjoy a good standard of living.

Dr. Tash was working on the wards as a fairly new consultant. He was very kind and had a caring, gentle bedside manner. Patients liked him although, in the opinion of his colleagues, his practice of medicine was mediocre. There were other physicians and surgeons who were very good doctors but often let down by their abrupt manner. Dr. Tash had an ingratiating manner and his patients, especially women, liked him.

Outside the medical ward, there were ancillary departments that ran a nine to five service, mainly doing tests for patients, such as ECGs (electrocardiograms) for tracing heart rhythms and vitalographs for testing the efficiency of the lungs. These departments were not locked as the ward might need to use them in emergencies.

At about seven one evening, I was returning some forms we had borrowed and I saw Dr. Tash carrying the vitalograph machine into the department. We said hello to each other and I thought no more of it. The following day I was talking to a junior doctor on the ward, and told him that I saw Dr. Tash with the machine.

"He'd just returned from a home visit to a private patient," the junior doctor replied.

"Oh," I remarked, wondering whether Dr.Tash had charged the patient for the use of the machine.

Later on I mentioned it to my nursing officer and she said it was fine to use the vitalograph as the wards wouldn't use it for emergencies, but he shouldn't borrow the ECG machine. It seemed that no one had ever challenged Dr.Tash for the unauthorised borrowing of the equipment, but the ward clerk overheard our conversation and remarked that Dr. Tash seemed to get away with quite a lot in the hospital. He was young and quite influential as a result of attending medical and management committee meetings.

On one occasion the ward clerk was having some blood tests done via Dr. Tash through her husband's private medical insurance and she didn't seem to be very happy about the way the tests were going.

"What happened?" I asked.

"Well, they lost the blood test that I had done last week. So much for the efficiency of private practice, and when I complained to Dr.Tash about it he didn't seem at all bothered and asked me to have another one done. He commented that it wouldn't cost me anything because the insurance firm would pay for it."

"Are you satisfied with that?"

"No, it means I shall have to undergo the discomfort and inconvenience of another blood test for which Dr.Tash will receive more money!"

Such was the temptation of money and the character of a doctor.

After two years in the medical ward I became the senior charge nurse in an acute surgical ward. A medical ward could be depressing because there could be six deaths in a weekend whereas the surgical ward was more volatile, with more routine admissions for smaller operations and patients were usually discharged quite quickly. We did, however, have some surgical patients in two side rooms, normally recovering from major operations such as arterial bypass, and some terminal patients receiving end-of-life care, but, on balance, it was a more cheerful ward.

In those days, we didn't have a private wing or facilities where only privately funded patients were treated and one day the telephone rang and I was asked by a junior doctor, who had been asked by Mr. Smilie, a surgical consultant, to move a terminal patient to the ward so as to allow his private patient to be admitted to a side room. I refused because the terminally ill patient was receiving many visitors and it seemed unfair to move a dying man to the main ward just because another patient could afford to pay for private treatment. Twenty minutes later my nursing officer came to the ward and informed me that Mr.Smilie had reported me for being "difficult to work with." I told her what had happened and the junior doctors felt that I was brave to stand up to the consultant.

"This is an NHS hospital, for all patients," I explained. "If there had been a side room available I would have given it to the private patient, but the care would be of the same high standard as it is for everyone else." The nursing officer couldn't convince me I was wrong, but she was able to find a side room in another ward in which to accommodate the patient.

Mr. Smilie appeared for the next ward round looking as smart as usual, wearing a bow tie and immaculate suit. We knew that he loved money and had not only a Mercedes but also a yacht. He warned me to "watch it" as I hadn't done as I was told.

During the ward round, he was discharging a patient with a large hernia. The patient was complaining about his in-growing toe nail which was very painful.

"I'll put you on a waiting list," Mr. Smilie said.

"How long is the waiting list?" asked the patient.

"Four months."

'But it hurts quite a lot.' The patient proclaimed.

"That is unless you want to go private," replied Mr. Smilie.

"How long would the waiting list be then?" the patient asked.

"I'll have you in next week."

"And how much would that cost?"

"Three hundred pounds," Mr. Smilie said.

In those days three hundred pounds was a lot of money.

"Oh, I'll have to think about that."

"Ok, let me know" said Mr. Smilie, walking away to see his next patient.

Such was the power of consultants and the attraction of money.

There were, however, many good consultants working in the NHS who would not take private patients. They were dedicated, extremely conscientious, and came to the wards to see their patients twice a day. They were well paid and treated every patient the same, regardless of their colour, sex, background or wealth.

That was in keeping with the founding principles of the NHS.

1979

Tale 7
Kay – A Mother's Tragedy

'*I must be cruel only to be kind.*' Wm. Shakespeare – Hamlet

In 1969, I was a senior charge nurse on an acute surgical ward. I was young, energetic and confident that doctors thought I was good at my job. I was willing to learn and always strived to be as efficient as I could. Like many nurses, I ate in the hospital canteen, where I was treated well and the staff always gave me a generous portion of food. I knew all the staff in the catering department and Kay, the catering manager, greeted me with a smile every time we met.

One of the most difficult jobs on the ward was giving patients and their relatives bad news. Mr. Franklin was a general surgeon. He was a small man, outspoken and quite trendy in his practice of medicine and surgery. He used to say that when he appeared to be cruel he was trying to be cruel to be kind. When a patient had advanced or terminal cancer, he always saw the relatives about the prognosis and, if the situation looked hopeless, he would explain the possible use of a "cocktail" of painkillers and sedation. It was unusual for a patient to survive three doses of this "cocktail" before fading peacefully away.

Tony was twenty-nine years old and a very sick young man. He was thin, drawn and looked quite ghastly although he had been ill only for four weeks. He was the son of Kay, the catering manager, and had recently had a scan which revealed a secondary cancer, originating from his stomach. Even worse, the cancer was spreading to his liver and he was in almost constant pain in spite of being given regular pain relief.

Mr. Franklin asked me to go to my office to discuss the situation. "Can you do me a favour, Patrick?" he asked.

"If I can," I replied.

Mr. Franklin and I got on well as a surgical team and he once said to me that if I was concerned about the performance of any of his junior doctors I should bypass them and discuss the matter with him. Such was the confidence of consultants in the ward sisters and charge nurses. Because the junior doctors came and went every six months and were mostly inexperienced, we were the most stable and trusted staff of the surgical team. We knew the routines and practices of medicine at least as well, and sometimes better than many of the junior doctors. The ward managers all felt good to be part of such an effective team.

"You know my house lady's work?" Mr Franklin continued.

I nodded, assuming he meant that her work was not of the best.

"And she doesn't speak English all that well! I wish I could remove her but I still have another four weeks to work with her."

The house lady was not very efficient at her work and was trying to do as little as possible.

"I have a difficult job I'd like you to do for me, Patrick. I would normally ask my house lady but I think you would do it better. I promised to see Kay about Tony's illness but I'm very busy this afternoon. Could you tell her the bad news for me please, and in two days time I'll talk to her in the outpatients department about my painkiller cocktail."

It was very difficult for me to turn down the request and I agreed to do it for him.

"Thanks Patrick, I owe you one," said Mr. Franklin.

I had seen relatives before to convey bad news, but not to someone I knew as well as I knew Kay. I was slightly nervous about it and at visiting time I gestured Kay over to the office.

"What do you think of Tony today, Kay?" I asked.

"I'm afraid he doesn't seem at all well," she replied.

I hesitated, not knowing quite how to break the awful news.

'Is it bad news, Patrick?'

I nodded, "I'm very sorry Kay to have to tell you that Tony has secondary cancer."

"Is it very bad?"

"I'm afraid so." I said, as kindly as I could. "Would you like a cup of tea?"

Kay nodded, looking down at the floor, looking hurt and bewildered. I made tea in the kitchen and brought it to her.

"What's the next step, Patrick?"

"Well, Mr. Franklin said he would talk to you in two days time, at two o'clock in the outpatients department."

"What will happen then, Patrick?"

"Well, you know that he is in a lot of pain."

"Yes, I just wish that he wasn't suffering."

"Well, Mr. Franklin will talk to you about more effective pain management that will help him."

"Thank you, Patrick," said Kay gratefully.

Tears were flowing down her face and I was speechless. As I touched her hand to show my sympathy I could feel tears in my eyes also. Kay sat in my office for another ten minutes to compose herself and then left.

Two days later, Kay saw Mr. Franklin and they agreed that Tony should be given the "cocktail". By then he looked so frail that his body was little more than a skeleton, a sight I was unable to banish from my mind for a long time. Even many years later I still remember it.

Tony's prognosis had been a very pessimistic one; at best he might live another month, if he was lucky, but after only two doses of the "cocktail" he died peacefully in his sleep. It is pointless to speculate why and how people so young and in the prime of life can so suddenly and fatally be stricken by such diseases, and impossible to imagine the effects of the death of a child on the parents.

A week or so later Kay sent us a box of chocolates in appreciation of the care we had given her son and fortunately, since then, I have not been called upon again to inform someone I knew about their dying child.

1978

Tale 8
Dr Lichfield and Dr Donovan – 1976

'Only the Good Die Young' Billy Joel

My first ward sister's post was on an acute medical ward where most of the ward sisters were female and the majority of them had been at the hospital for many years. The consultants seemed to get on well with them but, being the youngest ward sister on the medical unit, I was aware that I had to be efficient and professional in my work to earn their respect. Additionally, I was one of only two male charge nurses in the acute block.

The ward had four medical consultants, including Dr. Lichfield, a general physician, and Dr. Donovan who specialised in the treatment of diabetes. Dr. Lichfield was in his late fifties, rather old fashioned and very kind to patients. One of my main roles was to accompany consultants and their junior doctors on ward rounds. I had to be really on the ball to know exactly what was going on with their patients, for which Dr. Lichfield was always thankful. At times I knew more about the patients than the housemen, who had many wards to look after.

Dr. Lichfield had welcomed me to the ward when I started and I was grateful to him for that. I soon learnt his likes and dislikes, his procedures, methods of examining patients, and the fact that he liked to know the weight and ECG (electro-cardiogram) results of all his patients. To demonstrate my efficiency I always ensured that I had the latest results readily on hand. We got on well and I soon felt I was part of his team.

At Christmas time he was always generous and gave presents to all the trained staff, a mark of appreciation for all the work we had done throughout the year. Soon after one Christmas my nursing officer informed me that Dr. Lichfield was very ill and dying of a serious heart complaint. He advised me to look out for him as best I could. I was very sorry to hear how ill Dr. Lichfield was but I had noticed recently that he looked tired and exhausted after ward rounds. The following day, when I was with him during the ward rounds, I noticed that he had lost weight and his suit hung a little loosely on him. His face was pale and drawn, but he was working on as usual.

There were times when I wanted to ask a nurse to help me to sit a heavy patient up in bed for the consultant's examination, but Dr. Lichfield insisted on helping me himself and I felt very sorry to see him struggling. He was much older than me and I felt for him as if he were my father.

"Are you ok, Dr. Lichfield?" I asked anxiously on one occasion.

"Yes, I'm fine thanks."

"Would you like a cup of tea after your ward round?"

"No thanks, but it's very kind of you to offer."

I took a risk and asked a further question. "Why don't you have a rest and take some time off? You don't look well you know." It was not really my place to interfere and I must have shown my anxiety.

Dr. Lichfield was smiling. "Thanks for your concern, Mr. Poon, but I'm fine. I'd rather carry on with my work than stay at home brooding over my health."

"Take care then," I said.

Those were the last words I spoke to Dr. Lichfield. He died of a heart attack two days later, aged fifty-eight. Most of us went to his funeral service in the church on the hill in Walsall and we reflected on what life was all about.

He was such a good doctor, taken before his time, and all his skills and knowledge were buried with him in the ageless sands of time.

****

Dr. Donovan was a younger man of forty-two, a diabetic specialist who had been a consultant for five years. He was quite young for a consultant but right up-to-date and a very efficient doctor. I enjoyed his modern way of treating diabetes, especially for patients in a coma. His regime was acute, intense and efficient. We admired his work, although he was not an easy person to please and seemed to like finding fault with nurses.

He was very particular and focused much of his time on patients' medical charts. My other ward sister tried to avoid his ward rounds because she didn't like the comments he made following them, so I tried my best to cover his ward rounds, ensuring the charts and patients' results were all readily available. If they weren't Dr. Donovan could make life difficult. However, if the ward rounds were smoothly and efficiently conducted, he would be grateful and would thank you for your help.

He was a very committed doctor and if a patient of his was ill, he would go to the ward to see him or her twice or three times a day if necessary; something quite rare for a consultant. He was also very good with the relatives of patients. Rumour had it that before he used any new form of insulin injection for diabetic patients, he would try it on himself, even though he was not a diabetic. He wanted to know what it felt like to be the patient.

At Christmas time he would bring his two sons to the hospital, carrying a large box of chocolates and a bottle of wine for us. It was good to see him relaxing with his family and we shook hands and wished each other a happy Christmas.

In those days it was a tradition on the wards to ask a consultant to carve the turkey on Christmas day and the ward sisters used to agree amongst themselves who to ask to perform this task. Dr. Donovan was the consultant we asked most and he seemed to thoroughly enjoy the role.

The staff took a great pride in the ward at Christmas time. Decorations were put up, a Christmas tree stood in the corner and every member of staff did all they could to create a festive atmosphere in which the patients could enjoy themselves, in spite of their poor health.

Unfortunately, when spring arrived, we heard that Dr. Donovan was ill with cancer of the pancreas. He was a non-smoker, drank very little and ate sensibly. The world didn't seem to be fair to people who did so much to help others. We were surprised, however, when we heard he was advised to have a major operation to have the carcinoma removed, but he declined, and we wondered why. He carried on working while he was physically able to do so and because of his relatively young age, he was still alive the following Christmas. Although he was no longer working he popped onto the ward and I saw him in his suit and raincoat. He looked so jaundiced and haggard that I felt choked and upset.

"Hello, Dr Donovan, how are you keeping?" I said, trying to sound cheerful.

"So-so," he replied, smiling wryly. "It's Christmas time and I'm afraid didn't manage to buy the nurses' presents this year so here's a cheque for you. You can all go out and have a meal on me.'

I accepted the cheque for £50, which was a lot of money in those days. "Thank you very much, and a merry Christmas to you, Sir!"

I didn't normally called consultants sir, but he was looking so poorly and it was good of him to make such a generous gesture to us.

"Thank you for all your help, all of you, and goodbye," he said as he left the ward for the last time.

Two weeks later Dr. Donovan died and as we gathered at the church for his funeral service, we wondered why he had refused the operation. Did he know something we didn't, or was it the thought of the pain and discomfort he might suffer after the operation, for what might only be a temporary reprieve?

Looking back on my nursing career there have been no more deaths in service of doctors I have known and worked with. I continued working in hospitals as a senior nurse in two different hospitals for many more years and during that time it was usually retirement parties that I attended, but I often thought of the words of the Billy Joel song, "Only the Good Die Young" whenever I recalled the good deeds done by Dr. Lichfield and Dr Donovan.

Tale 9
Mr George and Mrs West's Shoplifting Spree

'Every true man's apparel fits your thief.' Wm Shakespeare.

I was a surgical charge nurse for two and a half years in an acute surgical ward. I was young, energetic and willing to learn. Work in the ward was hectic, exciting and rewarding. Turnover of patients was rapid and everyone, both doctors and nurses, worked highly efficiently. Most patients stayed on the ward for only a few days and were then discharged.

There were several consultants on the ward, including a urologist, arterial surgeon and general surgeons, performing all kinds of operations and they had house doctors working with them. House doctors were sometimes inexperienced, perhaps working on a surgical ward for the first time, and they often needed supervision. They came and went every six months and consultants relied on the nurses and surgical registrar to keep a watchful eye on them.

Ward sisters and surgical registrars were more experienced and were able to oversee the general routine work done for the patients by the house doctors.

There was a ward round every morning, conducted by a surgical registrar, to sort out bed vacancies for routine patients and to see which patients were ready for discharge. It was a very important role. Registrars usually stayed on the ward for one year or two. Some were very good at their job and others not so good.

Mr. George was a Chinese registrar from Malaysia. Both he and I could speak Cantonese but he was unable to read or write Chinese. He was well respected and was working on the wards as a house doctor before becoming a registrar. I was born in Hong Kong and occasionally we spoke to each other in Cantonese. We generally got on very well together.

Mr. George was an able surgeon and consultants were happy to leave him to perform most operations. The doctors and nurses seemed to like him too, as he was a quick, efficient worker who was also good and kind to relatives. He was a quiet man and kept himself to himself. No one knew very much about him but there was gossip in the hospital. It was said he had a wife in Hong Kong and an English girlfriend here in England, but his private life was no concern of ours. We listened, agreed his work was good and got on well together.

Off duty, I sometimes played tennis with him on the courts inside the hospital campus. We sometimes played singles and sometimes doubles with other doctors or nurses. After tennis we would engage in casual conversation, but never anything too deep or philosophical. He was a pleasant enough person, in his thirties, and, having worked in several hospitals, highly experienced.

On two occasions he rang me on the ward and asked me to lend him five pounds as he was short of money. I kept it to myself but thought it was strange that a registrar earning far more money than I did wanted to borrow from me. I lent him the money and he paid it back promptly. I wondered if the rumours were correct and that he did have one or two women in addition to his wife, but I never asked. I did once meet an English lady at a party, a ward sister from another hospital, and she and Mr. George seemed quite a couple.

He must have been working at the hospital for more than a year when he had his contract renewed. We were pleased as we all thought he was a nice fellow with good manners, and always kind to nurses. Consultants liked him too, and most important, he was a very able surgeon. It was pleasing for the ward staff because we all worked well in a closely-knit surgical team.

A few months went by and I was shocked to be told by a houseman that Mr. George's name was in the local newspaper, having been filmed by an in-store camera changing the price of a frozen chicken in a large supermarket. He appeared in court where he was found guilty and fined. We could never understand why he did this and dared not ask him, but we heard later that his contract had been terminated.

Before George left he told me that because he could speak Cantonese he was going to work in Hong Kong for a well- known private company. He left me a business card so that I could call him when I was Hong Kong the following year. I did call on him and we had lunch together. He was doing very well and earning lots of money as a surgeon. I also met his Chinese wife and we had pleasant afternoon together but we have not met since.

Three year after working as surgical charge nurse I was promoted to nursing officer of the surgical unit. The unit consisted of two general surgical wards, ear, nose and throat and a gynaecological ward. I worked there for five years and was in charge of some eighty nurses.

One afternoon, I was asked to go to the office of a senior nursing officer where I met a union steward from the Royal College of Nursing. I was informed that Mrs. West, one of my trained nurses, had been caught stealing from a supermarket. I was told that if the story got into the press she might lose her job because of her professional misconduct and the consequent bad publicity for the hospital. I was dumbfounded. Mrs. West was not a senior nurse but she was a very good one and it seemed she was in some financial difficulty.

Mrs. West and I never discussed the matter but fortunately no press reporters were present in court and the incident was not reported. To my relief, and no doubt hers, she was able to keep her job.

I often reflected deeply as to what it was that caused professional people, with well-paid jobs, to risk their reputations and livelihoods to save a few pence on the price of a frozen chicken or basket of groceries. Perhaps the risk of being found out gave them some kind of thrill? Did they not think of the implications?

Human nature and human behaviour is complicated and I didn't know the answers.

Tale 10
Anthony's Fortuitous Recovery

'*Cheer us when we recover: but let us pass on.*' Edmund Burke.

It was a warm and sunny Saturday and I was in town, just finishing my shopping. I was walking towards my car when a hand gently tapped my shoulder. I turned around and saw a sturdy young man with a black face and brown eyes.

"Hello, Mr. Poon. How are you?"

"Hello," I replied. His face was familiar and I tried to remember where I had seen him before.

"Can't you remember me?" he asked.

"I'm sorry, I know your face....."

"I'll give you a hint: your longest stay surgical patient," he said.

I smiled as recognition dawned. "Are you Anthony?"

"Yes, charge nurse Poon." His smile was friendly and welcoming.

"My word, you've grown, Anthony."

We gave each other a big hug, as if we were long lost friends.

"Well, well! It must have been three years," I said.

"No, Only two."

"You were so small then and you look so well and tall now."

Anthony smiled, "And you were all so good and friendly to me..........."

"What are you doing now?" I asked.

"I'm at college, studying engineering," Anthony replied.

"Great! I remember now. I did ask Mr. Sommerville how you were getting on some 18 months ago and he told me you were doing well."

I had a good look at Anthony and the satisfaction showed on my face.

"You are a Chinese and it's so easy to recognize you," Anthony declared.

"You're right, and I am so glad you tapped my shoulder, it's great to see you. You made my day."

"How is your surgical ward?" Anthony asked.

"As busy as ever, but it's always satisfying to help the sick."

"God bless all you nurses. You do such good job."

I nodded. Words couldn't express the feelings rekindled by this encounter. We shook hands and said goodbye.

Some two years previously I was a senior charge nurse and ward sister on an acute surgical ward. One day the telephone rang to say that I had to admit a little black boy from the children's ward. He was very small for a sixteen year old and he had a leaking abdominal fistula. He wouldn't normally be on a children's ward but he was there because he was unusually small for his age.

Two weeks previously he had a small operation on his abdomen to remove a rare kind of cyst and the wound hadn't healed properly. Fluid had been leaking continuously from

Anthony's abdomen since the operation and the surgeon, Mr. Somerville, was about to operate for a second time to assess what could be done to improve the situation. Anthony was gentle, softly spoken and looked very small on his adult bed. His family was poor and they could only visit him twice a week.

We prepared him for the exploratory operation and hoped it would be successful. The procedure went smoothly, no abnormality was detected, he recovered very well from the anesthetic and we started feeding him a soft diet. Unfortunately, the food wasn't digested properly and soon the wound was leaking again. Anthony was so dejected.

The following morning we had to change his dressing because it was soaked through. Anthony didn't complain even though it must have been uncomfortable and after we had changed the dressing we told the doctors what had happened.

The doctors discussed the matter with Mr. Somerville and Anthony's diet was reduced to soup and pudding, but it made no difference. The wound leaked so much that we had to change his dressing eight times in one day and he became so dehydrated that we had to put him on intravenous fluids. That worked well but we couldn't let him live on intravenous fluids for the rest of his life.

In the meantime the situation was explained to his family and they took the news well. Because of his age, we referred Anthony to a social worker and she arranged for an outreach tutor to teach him on the ward. He studied quite conscientiously but occasionally he became bored and homesick. He couldn't be discharged, even though he was physically well, because district nurses wouldn't be able to dress his wound eight times a day. Even so, Anthony seldom complained.

He liked helping us to give patients their mid-morning coffee, afternoon tea and evening drinks and the patients grew fond of him, but that was in 1980. Today, the service would be more impersonal and remote. The drinks would be served by the "hotel services" department and patients wouldn't be allowed to help at all.

Three months passed and it felt as if Anthony was becoming a permanent fixture, part of the furniture on a ward where patients usually stayed for less than a week. Occasionally, after a major operation, a patient might stay longer and some terminally ill patients might stay until they died, but a three month stay was exceptional. During those three months Anthony was only allowed to drink sips of water as most of what he ate and drank leaked out of his abdomen. It must have been very frustrating and we all felt very sorry for him.

The permanent nurses liked him and began to treat him almost as they would a member of staff. During their annual leave they would send him postcards and, when they returned, bring him small presents or souvenirs, but he remained small and his wound still leaked. We weighed him once a week but he gained no weight.

One day, a drug representative selling new products, saw Mr. Somerville, who was quite impressed with a product called clinifeed, a milk product which could be used as an intravenous transfusion. It was highly nutritious and Mr. Somerville decided to try it on Anthony, whose wound was sore with the frequent changing of the dressings. He was so fed up he would try anything.

The clinifeed drip worked wonders. Anthony's leak started

to dry up and he began to gain a little weight. For four and a half months he had only been able to drink sips of water and had tasted no solid food at all during that time. He was less than 17 years old, cheerful, uncomplaining and well-liked by everyone on the ward, but we all knew he must eventually be discharged to start a normal life, like any other seventeen year old.

Fortunately, clinifeed could be taken as a drink, like a thick liquid milk food, and Anthony was able to drink it although he didn't like it much. His dressing became drier and drier and he gained weight steadily. He was smiling and we were happy for him. After all this time, we wanted to help him to get back home to start living again. Hospital was no place to keep a youngster for so long.

Educationally, he was doing quite well but, sadly, his family was unable to visit him very frequently. Still, he remained cheerful and got on well with all the staff and patients on the ward. Jokingly, before he left, we awarded him the title of "The Longest Stay Model Surgical Patient."

We could hardly believe it. After 5 months he could eat and drink a little, with no side effects, and steadily gained weight. Mr. Somerville was very pleased and decided it was time for Anthony to go home.

When he was discharged, we felt there was a void on the ward. The helpful Anthony was gone. Two months later, I asked Mr Somerville how Anthony was doing and he told me that he was still improving. Nurses are a sentimental breed. We wouldn't pretend to be great heroes but we do care, and we enjoy helping people to improve their health and lives. We were pleased and proud to have played a part in Anthony's fortuitous recovery.

1980

Tale 11
Charge Nurse Colin's error – 1983

(*Errare humanum est* – Augustine of Hippo- Sermons 164:14) –To err is human

To err is human? Colin was a senior charge nurse (equivalent to the grade of a ward sister) of an ear, nose and throat ward. He ran the ward very well, usually with shrewd expertise, tremendous skills and wide and profound knowledge in the specialties of ear, nose and throat. He was trained in the Army, hence, he always dressed immaculately and constantly present himself for being helpful.

The operations on ear, nose and throat were relatively small scale and short by nature but there were usually numerous to be done in one session. In a morning, the ward would 'do' more than10 operations such as tonsillectomies.

Staff and nurse and tutors liked Colin. Each operation might take 15 minutes. Hence, there were many on the list one morning for a four hours session. Nurses on the same ward were capable also. The doctors liked them and they got on very well. One 'operating' morning about 10.30, my bleep went. It was operating theatre. They wanted to see me. I went to theatre and saw the Nursing Officer there.

He told me,' Sorry to tell you this, Patrick, we nearly

operated on a wrong patient, if the theatre end did not check it properly!'

'What??' I could not believe what I was hearing.

Checking the correct patient for the correct procedure was a fundamental but very important procedure. One staff usually checked the right case note, the unit number, and name of patient and date of birth against the arm bracelet wormed by the patient. No matter how many patients we were to operate on.

'Who checked it on the ward?' I demanded.

'Colin.' I could not believe my ears.

'I will sort it out.' I said.

The wrong patient, a little boy, was sent back to the ward, re-waiting for his turn.

In the ward, Colin was waiting for me, looking embarrassed.

'What is happening, Colin?' I was not happy.

'I am sorry, Patrick, I do not know what happened. The telephone rang and someone else asked me about something else and I thought I had checked and followed the procedure also.....'

'But you did not check it thoroughly!' I asserted.

'I have to own up, it was my fault.' Colin sighed.

'Good job the theatre checked it properly; otherwise we will be in big trouble! Have you any thought for the patient, his parents/guardians; the press?' I admonished.

'I know, I know, I am sorry and I plead guilty. I have never done this before.' Colin was looking unhappy too.

'Are you having any problems at home?' I enquired humanely.

'No, I am fine. It is just one of those things.' He sheepishly proclaimed.

'But someone nearly had a wrong operation!' I admonished again.

'I know.' He retorted as he looked toward the floor as if it could open up to swallow him in a single gulp.

'Sorry, Colin, I have to report this. Theatre knows, everybody knows.'

'I know.' He further dipped his head in anguish.

The official complaint procedure started as Colin could not explain the reason. My seniors were informed. Because of Colin's good track record, he was given a final warning for a year. Final warning was given because of the seriousness of the matter. If he did it again within a year, his position would be terminated. What a blessing it was checked and caught by theatre staff! Otherwise, one could not imagine what could have been done wrong to a right patient! How come Colin slipped up? Was he stressed? Problems at home? No one knew.

****

Sometimes, a very good staff would still make mistake. In another instance, Staff nurse John did a similar thing. On a very busy surgical ward, he checked some blood transfusion with a student nurse; wrong blood was put up to the correct patient. Fortunately, it was found out 15 minutes later and the transfusion was immediately stopped and the patient was reasonably unaffected and doctors informed. Again, the proper procedure has not been followed through.

This incident also transpired that later the usually competent staff's nurse received a first written warning. Fortunately, for Colin and John, both were given the warnings and it was for one year. After one year, once their performance was clear and no further reoccurrence. They would have their warnings rescinded. However, it was a horrible time for the staff and the patients.

*

At the corner of my desk, there were some books about nursing and medicine. One of them was an annual report book on surgical nursing from a nursing association. One report informed us the past year, there were 10 wrong limbs removed in the operating theatres in England, some legs and arms have been amputated wrongly, the left kidney was removed instead of the right kidney were some irreversible blunders. I was appalled by such reports.

To err is human but these checking procedures in hospitals are vital standard because many a time the mistake(s) could not be remedied or corrected. How could wrong limbs have been marked by doctors and patients have been operated on? How could wrong patients have been checked clear to proceed in the operating theatre?

There were at least two strict procedures to check to ensure correct patients were having the operations. One was at the ward and the other one at the entrance of the theatre. Hospitals were very busy places and many staff at work but all these procedures were done so many times a day and it must be checked and double checked thoroughly.

Tale 12
Larry's Nightmare – 1993

'*Dreams are true while they last.*' Alfred, Lord Tennyson

Larry was a very good and caring health care assistant on the Ear, Nose and Throat ward. He was hard working, willing to learn and always helpful. Patients and staff all liked him. Even doctors spoke highly of him, of his care for the patients and of his endearing personality. Several times I overheard him reassuring apprehensive patients before entering theatre and they sometimes asked him if he could wait for them until they came back. Larry, being the caring and conscientious person he was, would invariably be there. It is no wonder he passed his NVQs with flying colours and was soon accepted for nurse training. Everyone was expecting him to be a committed, competent and reliable staff nurse within a few years.

I was an operational officer and my duties included being on call, a week at a time, one week in every four. Nurses on call covered all kinds of problems, twenty-four hours a day for seven days. It could be stressful and sometimes involved finding solutions to difficult problems. Even then, we did not have enough beds for patients and at times I would take a call in the early hours of the morning, asking me to find a bed for a sick child.

One evening when I was on call, Debbie, a trained nurse called me at home.

"Mr. Poon, I'm sorry to ring you at home."

"Not to worry, Debbie."

This was the first time I had been called by Debbie. She was an intelligent, highly competent and experienced nurse. Something serious must have happened.

"What's wrong, Debbie?" I asked.

"It's difficult to tell you on the 'phone" she replied, "Can you come in?"

"No problem, Debbie, I'll see you in fifteen minutes."

In the ward office, Debbie looked puzzled, slightly anxious and not her usual self.

"Don't worry, Debbie, just tell me what it is," I said reassuringly.

"Well, you know Larry, everybody likes him and he's such a good carer."

"Yes, I agree. He has a very good reputation. So, what happened?"

"Mr. Smith is an overnight case," she explained, "he'd just had his operation, everything was fine and he's due to go home tomorrow."

"Good, please go on," I said.

"But his wife has just been to see me. She said Larry brought her husband back from the operating theatre and as he put him back to bed and made him comfortable, Larry was acting in a strange and inappropriately 'playful' manner. In fact, she said he was playing with her husband's penis."

"Never!" I replied, "That's a very serious accusation and I find it difficult to believe of Larry."

"Well, I'm afraid that's what she said and I have no reason to disbelieve her," said Debbie. "Mr. Smith is obviously very concerned and upset. He told his wife what had happened and she has been to see me."

"It does seem completely out of character, but if it's true the consequences for Larry could be very grave indeed."

"Exactly, that's why I rang you."

"You haven't said anything Larry then?"

"No, it's very difficult to know how to approach it."

"I just can't believe it," I said. "It just doesn't seem right."

We both thought of Larry as a good, caring and thoroughly reliable person and we couldn't imagine him doing such a thing so I decided to telephone the on-call nursing director for advice. He couldn't believe that Larry could be so stupid as to do such a thing either, but said I should suspend him on full pay pending a full investigation.

I telephoned the ward sister, Ann, and told her what had happened. She could understand why we had to suspend Larry but still found it very difficult to believe the allegation. As Larry had gone off- duty, Sister and I made arrangements to see him the following morning.

The following day I saw Mrs Smith, the wife of the patient, and explained that there was a formal procedure we had to follow and later that morning Sister and I asked to see Larry in the office. As I outlined the allegation that had been made against him the colour drained from his cheeks as if he had been confronted by a ghost and he said he couldn't believe what I had told him.

"I am sorry, Larry." I said, "I can't believe it either, but it is a very serious allegation and we have to discover the truth."

"But I only brought him back from theatre and got him out

of the stretcher," explained Larry. "The theatre orderly helped me and then I just took off his theatre gown and changed him into pyjamas."

"We believe you Larry, Sister said, but you do understand that we have to investigate the incident and then explain to Mrs Smith why her husband said what he did."

I had never seen a person so hurt and upset. Larry's face was the colour of faded parchment and I could see he was trying to hold back the tears.

"Larry, I'm very sorry but we have to suspend you until further notice, on full pay, a procedure that the hospital has to follow." Sister and I looked at each other with sadness and without another word Larry packed his bag and left.

Soon after, I went to the operating theatre and told Dr. Andy, the head anaesthetist, what had happened. He was quite calm and asked to see the case notes. I handed them over and he checked to see what anaesthetic had been used for Mr. Smith's operation.

"Yes, that is what I thought," Dr. Andy said.

"What is that? Is it the drug you used?" I asked.

"Yes, it is. The anaesthetic I used has at least a 10% chance of giving patients erotic dreams."

"What! Why don't we inform the patients before anaesthetising them?'

"Well, all the drugs we use have side effects, you know."

"But poor Larry's terribly upset and shocked by the allegation."

"I think you should have a word with him as soon as he comes back." Dr. Andy replied. "You're the nursing director so you should see him first and I'll see him afterwards. Then I'll speak to the patient and his wife, explain to them exactly what happened and reassure them that I have no doubt that it was a reaction to the anaesthetic that caused Mr Smith to say what he did. I'll assure her that the alleged incident took place only in her husband's imagination."

"That's fine," I said, "but it seems so unfair to Larry."

"Well, unfortunately we can't explain every possible side-effect of every drug we use."

I tried to ring Larry to inform him of the conversation I had with Dr. Andy in the operating theatre but he didn't answer the phone. I asked the ward sister to telephone him but there was still no answer. We knew Larry was very deeply hurt and we also felt quite upset about the incident.

The explanations given by the anaesthetist and director of nursing to the patient and his wife were not as well-received as we had hoped. They thought it was an attempt at a cover-up, but the senior staff of the hospital explained again that what had happened was a well- known side-effect of that particular anaesthetic and stressed that if Mr and Mrs Smith were not happy with the answer they could take their complaint further. After some thought and reflection they decided to accept the explanations given to them. The effect of this unfortunate event made the atmosphere in the ward quite uncomfortable. What was going on? Where was Larry and why was he not at work? Because the events that had taken place were confidential, we were unable explain every detail of what had happened.

We wrote to Larry and invited him to come to the hospital to meet the senior doctor and ward sister who explained to him that it was not his fault at all. Larry was reinstated without a stain on his character and returned to work but he seemed quiet and withdrawn. He asked for a transfer to a job that didn't involve intimate nursing procedures and his request was granted, but sadly he left the wards shortly afterwards and never became a student nurse.

Some years later, I left the NHS and went into further education where I taught NVQ levels 2, 3 and 4. One of the mandatory units was "Abuse, its Effects and Implications." I often quoted Larry's case of alleged sexual abuse, an allegation which proved to have no basis in fact, but which ended his chosen career. It was both unfortunate and unfair. I felt sad that a young man's potentially good nursing career had been destroyed before it had really started.

I didn't see him again until about ten years later. I was walking down the street when I felt a tap on the shoulder. I turned around and there was Larry. He was chatty and friendly, just as he was in the old days, before the incident. Both of us looked older, and perhaps wiser. We didn't speak about the incident but his kindly gesture, after all those years, filled me with a sense of relief and calm. He was still working in the hospital, but in a different department, testing patients on hearing monitors. I was pleased to hear he was doing well and enjoying his job and somehow, I felt a sense of closure.

God bless you, Larry.

Tale 13
Inquest – Accidental Death

'Advice is seldom welcome and those who want it like it least,'
P.D. Stanhope

I had been a surgical nursing officer for two years, not the easiest of jobs because I was "in the middle" between ward sisters and senior officers. I was no longer attached to a particular ward but I was gradually becoming accustomed to the change of role and, one day, I received a call advising me to be ready for an inquest into Mr. Hogan's death.

I vaguely remembered the case. Mr Hogan had died after a fall on one of my surgical wards about nine months previously. I was on duty on the evening it happened, and having checked the records to see who was on duty on the ward in question, I discovered it was staff nurse Ray. I read the old case notes and noted that Mr. Hogan was recovering from a stomach operation and was restless. He was 72 years old, rather stubborn and wouldn't listen to advice. He was asked to sit still in the dayroom but refused. He tried to stand up and walk about, fell down and broke his femur. He needed an urgent operation and his relatives were informed. After an emergency operation he was transferred to an orthopaedic ward and he died shortly afterwards.

An inquest must be held in respect of any death happening within 48 hours after an operation and it was arranged to be held in the hospital. I talked to staff nurse Ray, who recalled the incident. He had filled in the accident book, as required, in the presence of a student nurse and his recollection of the facts coincided with the record in the case notes. Ray, who had qualified only six months previously, asked me for my advice but I confessed that it was my first inquest and advised him to just truthfully relate the facts.

I searched the ward records and found that the normal quota of four staff were on duty on the evening in question. Ray recalled that it was not a very busy evening. Mr. Hogan was indeed asked to sit still, refused, stood up, tried to walk and fell. Relatives were informed.

Because I was apprehensive I asked my boss and colleagues if they could give me any advice, but none of them had been to an inquest and I was just advised to tell the truth. Fortunately, the records were clear and precise. I could find no omissions or mistakes, and I gathered all the information I thought was relevant. Neither Ray nor I had any advice or assistance from anyone and as a result, we were both quite nervous.

If the incident happened today, people being much more aware of the legal consequences of such events, I wondered whether we would have been given some assistance. No one at the hospital had offered to help and no one had advised us to approach the College of Nursing, of which we were both members. We were simply left to get on with it alone.

The inquest was rather like a trial. The chairman asked Ray to give his rank and job-title and to explain what happened that evening. Ray answered honestly, describing what had happened and confirming that all the necessary procedures were carried out and all requirements fulfilled. He was asked if he was so rushed off his feet that he ignored the patient and he explained that it was a relatively quiet evening, but the patient did not accept the advice given to him. He stood up, tried to walk around and fell over. There was a reporter at the inquest and he wrote down all the facts in his notebook.

When it was my turn, I had to stand up and answer questions asked by the coroner. I was asked if the ward was understaffed and I replied that we normally had four staff on duty on that ward and that was how it was on the evening in question. I explained my role in the hospital and confirmed that the staff nurse on the ward had followed the correct procedure and that nothing untoward had happened. It was an ordeal, but fortunately we survived it. We thought the inquest went well and it was a relief that we weren't accused of any malpractice.

Whether it was an oversight by the hospital senior officers I don't know, but we had no formal feedback from anyone about the accident or the result of the inquest. For staff nurse Ray and me, it was a nerve-wracking experience because we had no one to consult with properly. Perhaps I should have been more persistent in asking for advice but no one had appeared at an inquest before. Today there would be a Human Resources Department to consult, with experience of legal tribunals and claims for compensation, and I feel that the matter would be treated much more seriously. I was not sure that in 1983 the personnel department knew anything about the inquest, or whether it was regarded as just a nursing matter to be dealt with by senior nurses. It was certainly an unusual experience.

1983

Tale 14

My Mistakes

'The cautious seldom err ...' Confucius.

We all make mistakes, so we are told, but in nursing patients' lives are at stake and we had to be very careful. I was an extremely careful man and checked things repeatedly, almost obsessively, but still I made mistakes.

In the 70s and 80s, doing drug rounds and giving out drugs was a long process, especially in the mornings and evenings on a medical ward. Every patient was on some kind of medication, but the interruptions we had were endless because, being a ward sister, I was the only one who had the latest information as to what was going on. There were telephone inquiries from doctors, relatives and pharmacies and it wasn't unusual to take three hours to complete one drug round.

One morning, I discovered that I had given twice the prescribed dose of valium to a patient. I couldn't explain why or how this happened and confessed to the house doctor. He wasn't too concerned as the worst that could happen was that the patient would have to sleep it off. It could have been worse.

Once or twice a month, usually in the afternoon, we had someone admitted as an outpatient to have a pint or two of blood drained off, because they suffered from polycythaemia, a condition where a person produces too many red blood cells. The patient would have a blood test so we knew his haemoglobin result and the doctor would decide how much blood to drain off.

The houseman had inserted the needle and I arranged an intravenous set upside down to drain off the blood. It should have been checked after half an hour but the interruptions and telephone calls from doctors and others made me forget the patient. By the time I remembered, I had drained off 500ml more than I should have. My heart nearly stopped but thankfully the patient was looking fine. I was feeling panicky and informed the houseman. I was assured that it would be fine as the patient was full of red blood cells. We checked the blood again and it was within normal limits. I felt bad about it and apologised to the patient who had been in my care several times previously. He was very nice about it but it worried me so much that I resolved never to let it happen again.

I always got on well with the junior doctors, perhaps because we were of a similar age or because I didn't normally nag them to do their work. One houseman told me that if I bleeped him, he knew it meant that I needed him whereas some ward sisters bleeped him, sometimes repeatedly, when he wasn't really needed.

I sympathised for the junior doctors, especially at weekends, when they were on call from 9 o'clock on Saturday morning until the following Monday morning. It was quite common for them to have very little sleep for two or three nights. In those days we had trolleys delivered to the wards for us to serve the meals and I would save some food for the doctors because sometimes they were so busy with emergency admissions they hadn't had time to eat, perhaps for up to eighteen hours.

On Monday mornings I often pleaded with the consultants doing the ward rounds to go easy on the doctors because they had probably not slept for two or three nights. The replies from the consultants were normally something like, "Well, they're young and they'll be fine," or "well, I did that in my early days and now it's their turn!" Sympathy from the senior doctors was rare.

On one occasion a surgeon had to relent and send a junior doctor to bed because he fell asleep at the operating table while holding the retractors. He hadn't slept for three nights. Although I was sometimes told off by senior doctors for interfering with medical staffing, I knew they respected me for supporting them. I worried as to what might happen to the patients if junior doctors made mistakes because they were so tired.

Many years later the General Medical Council decided to reduce junior doctors working hours as they were unsafe. Newspaper reports indicate that doctors have been killed in car crashes on Monday mornings while returning exhausted from a very busy weekend.

I had been a senior ward sister for three years and my superior, the nursing officer, was about to retire. On her recommendation I applied for her job and, following an interview, I was offered the post. I was told that, at thirty-one, I was the youngest nursing officer in general nursing in the Midlands.

I found being accountable for four wards, rather than one, very different but I was working in the wards where I was once a charge nurse and knew the staff well. They were all very good, hard working, caring and supportive.

One day, the ward sister of the surgical ward informed me that the trained nurse Pearl had admitted that she had injected twice the required dose into a T tube to a gallbladder. She was honest enough to admit the mistake as she did not wish to harm the patient but the houseman said it would be fine and the patient would not be harmed. The drug would merely be secreted through the urine.

I knew the ward sister was the most caring of nurses and yet this had happened. Officially I should file a report and she would be reprimanded, pending a full investigation, but I was reluctant to do that because she was such a good nurse. If I failed to file the report and was found out, I would be in trouble also. Should I be ruthless and take the official route, or should I overlook it?

That evening I went to the ward purposely to talk to the patient's consultant. He was the senior doctor of the ward and a nice man, but he was also a member of the senior management team. Nurses liked him too, but he might not be on the nurse's side. I met him, explained what had happened and he confirmed what the houseman had said, "The patient will be ok, no harm has been done and Pearl is such a good nurse, you shouldn't take it any higher."

"Thank you, I thought the same," I replied.

"Sometimes, we have to be kind to nurses." He smiled, winked and shook hands.

On reflection, I was taking a risk for a nurse I didn't want to lose. Officially, I should have reported the incident but it would have adversely affected a good nurse. Did I make a mistake or not? I don't know, but I was pleased I did what

I did. Pearl was very pleased and thanked me and the ward sister for our support. It was good to see humanity sometimes in some doctors!

1978

Tale 15

Staff Nurse Jane obeys orders

'Thus one who lacks courage cannot help others.' Daisaku Ikeda

Weekends were normally very busy in an acute general hospital. Emergency patients of all specialties were admitted; heart attacks, drunks and overdoses. As a nursing officer one of the problems I dreaded was the shortage of beds. Patients were sometimes put wherever there happened to be a bed, irrespective of the specialties. Doctors could put a medical patient on an acute surgical ward, for instance, or an asthmatic could be put on a general surgical ward where patients were recovering from operations. Many issues were raised because the essential medical equipment might not be available on a surgical ward and many meetings between doctors and senior nurses were held to discuss the best ways of putting patients on appropriate wards.

One Saturday morning staff nurse Jane telephoned me from the surgical ward. "Mr. Poon, Dr. Taylor wants to put an overdose patient on my ward. I told him that we were not allowed to as we are on the first floor, but he insisted because other medical patients were too ill to be on a surgical ward. He assured me that it would be ok. I'm not really happy with it. What do you think?"

I told her I would enquire whether there were any beds anywhere on the ground floor and that I would call her back. All the beds on the ground floor were full and I told staff nurse Jane, who told me that Dr. Taylor had been to the ward to say the overdose patient would be ok there. Everyone was under pressure with the acute shortage of beds that day.

On Sunday morning at about 9.00 I asked Jane if the patients were ok and she said they were, including the female overdose patient, although she did seem withdrawn and quiet. She was to be seen by a psychiatrist the following day.

At 10.30 a distraught Jane rang me again. "Mr. Poon, come to the ward quickly please. The overdose patient has broken the window and jumped to the ground. She's lying on the yard."

I didn't go to the ward immediately but to the ground floor to see to the patient, who was in pain, motionless and quiet. The porters came and we carried her carefully to a trolley and I wondered whether she had broken her back. Doctors were administering analgesics and ordering X-rays. I went to the ward and found staff nurse Jane sobbing and blaming herself not being strong enough to stand up to Dr. Taylor. She was highly stressed and became quite hysterical. I tried to reassure her, saying it was not her fault at all, but to no avail. On the corridor, I met Dr. Taylor and told him what had happened, and about the state Jane was in. He looked embarrassed and went to apologise to Jane but this did nothing to relieve her anxiety.

The patient was x-rayed and it was found that her lumbar spine was broken, a serious but not life-threatening injury. This was explained to her relatives and they took the news well. The patient was transferred for specialist treatment to an orthopaedic hospital some thirty miles away, where she was successfully operated on, but remained immobile for a long time.

Staff nurse Jane remained very upset and, having tried in vain to pacify her, I suggested that she should go home to relax. She eventually accepted the offer but was off sick for three weeks with severe stress, still blaming herself for the incident. Fortunately she recovered completely and returned to work on the ward.

The senior managers took the incident no further, other than to introduce a policy preventing any overdose patient being admitted to a first floor ward. If the policy had been introduced earlier both the overdose patient and Jane would have been spared a considerable amount of pain and stress.

The nightmare of bed shortages remained. Wards were used to accommodate both sexes, ignoring the privacy and dignity of patients. Beds could be found in corridors and patients could wait on hard trollies in casualty for hours. Patients with different specialties could be found on any ward in the hospital.

Since then the number of available beds has been further reduced and, like a black hole, there seems to be no known solution to the eternal problem.

1989

Tale 16
Help in the air

'A man must trust his feelings.'

One Saturday afternoon I was on duty from 1.00pm until 8.30pm, not a pleasant evening shift. Dr. Tash, the medical consultant, was on call and he called in to see if we had any problems. It was good of him to do that as we didn't often see him during the weekend.

"Any problems on the ward?" he asked.

"No thanks Dr. Tash. Have you heard about the accident near the Arboretum?" The Arboretum was our local park.

"Yes." He hesitated. "I heard many people were hurt near there. Several cars were involved, I understand."

"Yes, quite a few."

"Did you help?" A student nurse asked, rather unwisely.

"Well, no, I didn't want to get involved in any legal issues," Dr. Tash replied.

"Oh," the student was surprised that a nearby consultant didn't offer to help.

"Well, sometimes, we have to be very careful," I interjected.

Dr. Tash didn't want to get involved in a long discussion and left the ward.

"I would have stayed and helped," the student said, "wouldn't you, Patrick?"

"Yes, I would, especially since there were so many people involved."

We remained silent, not wishing to continue the conversation.

The legal and ethical issues were blurred. There had been instances reported in the newspapers where someone had offered help and been rewarded with someone suing them. It was not a black and white matter.

However, I felt there were certain situations where one had no choice but to help.

Once, I was flying from England to Hong Kong, my homeland. It was a long flight and I was trying to relax by reading a book when I was disturbed by an announcement. "If there is a doctor on board would you please raise your hand as we should appreciate your assistance." I looked around and didn't see anyone raising their hand. Being a trained nurse, I was wary and not sure whether I should offer to help or not, especially as they had asked for a doctor. The announcement was repeated, but still no one came forward.

Fifteen minutes later there was another announcement. "Is there a nurse on board? If so we would appreciate your help please."

Once again I looked around and didn't see a hand raised. An air stewardess went by and I stopped her. "I'm a trained nurse, is there a problem?"

"Yes, please come with me and help us, if you would," she replied.

I followed her upstairs to a man travelling first class. His nose was bleeding profusely and a male steward was trying unsuccessfully to help. Blood stained tissues were everywhere.

"I'm a nurse, can I help?" I asked.

"This nose bleed won't stop and I'm worried," the passenger said. He looked frightened and quite pale.

I turned to the steward, "OK, could you fetch me some ice and a small towel please?"

The steward brought the ice which I wrapped in the towel, placed it on the passenger's nose and I pinched the top of his nose very hard.

"This will be uncomfortable," I warned him.

The passenger nodded and tried to relax.

After fifteen minutes of really firm pressure on the blood vessel, the nosebleed subsided and the passenger and I were both relieved.

"You work in general nursing?" the passenger asked.

"Yes, I'm a male ward sister in an acute hospital but I did work in casualty for a year," I replied.

"Thank goodness," he said.

I stayed with him for a further five minutes until he was completely recovered and went back to check on him twenty minutes later. He was looking much happier and shook my hands to thank me again. I advised him to have his blood pressure checked by his general practitioner as soon as possible and returned to my seat feeling satisfied that my intervention had been successful. When I was leaving the plane I heard someone say that it was reassuring to have a medical person on board.

Several years later another incident took place, once

again on a flight to Hong Kong. The whole sequence of announcements and requests for help was repeated and because there was no response I offered to help again. An air stewardess was lying on the floor, in pain and pregnant. She asked my advice as to whether she should take more analgesics, having taken a strong pain kiiler only an hour before. I advised her not to. It was a simple answer and any doctor or nurse would have given the same advice.

It feels good to be able to help a person in need, especially when no one else is able to help but the possible legal implications did cross my mind. If my intervention had done more harm than good might I end up being sued for negligence?

But there is a very satisfying side to helping people. To be able to relieve pain and help to make people feel better must be one of the nicest feelings in the world.

1970

Tale 17
A Volunteer translator

'Our strength lies in our capacity for empathy with others.'

In the 1980s, when I was working as an operational manager in a hospital surgical unit, the staff were all asked if they would like to do some volunteer work as translators for patients in the south Staffordshire area. Some doctors volunteered for the French language and some for the language of their native country. I was born in Hong Kong and could speak Cantonese fluently so I volunteered. The following is my story.

My first assignment was to translate for a Chinese woman, Huan. The request came from a community psychiatric nurse who found it difficult to assess Huan's situation properly, because her husband was reluctant to talk. The problem came to light when a health visitor went to the Huan's home. She had recently given birth, and was depressed. The home was unusually untidy and Huan seemed to be isolated, distant, and neglecting herself.

I had to drive some twenty miles to the meeting and the psychiatric nurse had to remind Huan's husband to drive his wife to the appointment. I learnt more of the case history while I was waiting for them to arrive. Huan had only been in Britain for three years, in which time she had two children. She spoke no English, couldn't drive and an old photograph indicated she had aged considerably.

Like many Chinese in England, her husband was a chef. He also liked to gamble, which made his wife unhappy. She was given £50 a week for her and the children to live on, not very much at all. Her husband was hoping to open a Chinese take away, but so far had made little progress.

I told the community nurse that this was a familiar story, a Chinese person on foreign soil, lonely and with language problems. She lived in Lichfield, a small city in the Midlands, and a universe away from the bustling streets of Hong Kong. I felt that she was homesick, and had no one to talk to, especially in Cantonese. I remembered feeling like that myself, many years ago.

I wasn't surprised that the couple didn't turn up for the appointment. With me there, the husband wouldn't be able to control the translation. When the nurse telephoned the family, the husband said he had forgotten the appointment, although he was reminded of it two days previously. I felt helpless, frustrated and sad. He didn't want to sort out the problems at all. It was easier to escape into silence, especially if speaking the truth left you vulnerable.

Another time, I was interpreting in a hospital for a woman with diabetes, who had just lost a leg. Naturally, she wanted to know the reason and what the future held for her. The doctors asked me to help because her children, who were interpreting for her, knew that their mother was terminally ill and didn't want to tell her. They wouldn't tell her why she was in so much pain, why she had the operation, or what the treatment the doctors were giving her was designed to accomplish. They just wanted to protect her.

In another case, I was asked to interpret for a speech therapist who was helping two boys with problems. It wasn't just a matter of lacking confidence in a bilingual environment. There were real development problems which needed to be addressed, but when the boys were tested their mother would provide them with the correct answers, so no one would know how bad the problems were. I was needed as an impartial observer, who would interpret the responses accurately. Once this was done, the therapist was able to obtain the information she needed and the boys were on the road to recovery.

Unfortunately the outcome for homesick Huan was not so happy. There was little I could do, except give the address of a Birmingham Chinese Community to the nurse, to give to Huan, in the hope that she might be able to find a Chinese companion at some point. What else could I do if others didn't want to know?

On the way home, I felt a sense of nothingness. It was raining heavily, the sky was dark and for lonely Huan a beautiful dream had turned into a nightmare. All there was left were feelings of loss, despair and silence.

1990

Tale 18
Unusual Situations

'Flocks of the memories of the day draw near.' Alice Meynell

Some situations and patients stick in one's mind for many years. While writing this collection of memories, many things I thought I had forgotten came back to me. A long-forgotten name or event would suddenly come back to me with a vivid clarity. Some of the memories were happy, others painful and here are a few of the most unusual.

i) A cucumber in the rectum.

One afternoon, I was working on a surgical ward as a charge nurse, when I received a telephone call from the admission room asking us to prepare a bed for a sick patient. He was going to the operating theatre to have a cucumber removed from his rectum, the result, he said, of a violent quarrel. It was a very unusual situation. The man was in shock and it was thought that his peritoneum, a membrane covering most organs of the body, might have been perforated. If that was the case, it could cause peritonitis, which might be fatal. The police were involved but they were asked to come back the following day. On return from the theatre, the patient, who was pale but satisfactory, had an intravenous infusion. The cucumber had been completely removed and the damage to the peritoneum was only slight. A nasogastric tube was inserted to drain off any fluids from the stomach as a precaution.

The patient was a strong man. He recovered well and was discharged within a week. He was acutely embarrassed by the situation as the quarrel began over something very small and ended up in a heated fight. Fortunately, the operation was promptly done and saved the patient's life.

The following day, the Police arrived to take a statement and the attacker was subsequently arrested and charged with assault, causing actual bodily harm.

ii) Baby in the admission room.

When I first became a nursing officer, I was in charge of four surgical wards and an admissions room which was used for patients temporarily admitted to assess whether they needed medical or surgical admissions, or whether they could be discharged. I sometimes helped with the work there when the nurse was very busy.

Late one morning, we were told to expect an admission for a baby and I was not happy as the department was hardly equipped to look after babies. The baby should have been sent straight to a ward, to be seen by the paediatric doctor and nurses but they were very busy and didn't have an empty bed. On arrival, the baby was so cyanosed (literally meaning "the blue disease") and could hardly breathe. We found a very small catheter and connected it to an oxygen cylinder.

We called a doctor, who came immediately, and the baby's

hearted stopped. We sounded the cardiac arrest button and many doctors arrived on the scene. All the standard procedures were started but the baby died, in spite of all the doctors there trying their best to save the baby. The crying of the mother penetrated through the corridor. I was very inexperienced in children's nursing, hadn't dealt with child patients for many years and had never before held a dead baby.

The mother was still holding the baby when, fortunately, my colleague, a highly experienced paediatric nursing officer arrived. She consoled the mother, offered to hold the baby in her arms and took them to a side room where they wouldn't be disturbed.

The scene is still embedded in my memory. The nursing officer was holding the baby as if it were her own. It was a relatively small gesture, but to me the act was very kind and almost holy. It made me appreciate the skills of specialist medicine and nursing; the care of children, gynaecology, surgical, medical and cardiac nursing

I thanked my colleague for helping the nurse and me. She told me that the baby should not have gone to the admissions room and said she would ensure this didn't happen again.

iii) Status epilepticus.

Epilepsy affects between 40 and 70 people per 100,000 people annually and the condition is treated and controlled by medication. My nursing career started in 1968 in a psychiatric hospital in Hong Kong and it was there I first saw epileptic patients. Some of them were children who were categorised as GPI, meaning general paralysis of the insane, a term we very rarely come across now. It was caused by syphilis, a disease transmitted by sexual intercourse with several partners. We had a few patients suffering from the disease and we were warned not to touch their blood and to ensure we didn't have an open wound, otherwise we could be infected via the blood contact. In those days, we didn't even wear gloves when giving patients an injection.

Patients suffering from GPI, and their children, tended to be epileptics and we were taught how to look after them when fitting. It was an unpleasant sight when one saw it for the first time. It often started with a noise and the patient would start shaking or convulsing, with limbs jerking and eyes rolled up. Muscles were contracted and the patient would fall to the ground. The body would fit or shake for minutes but soon the patient would relax and the muscles would loosen. Very often, the relaxation caused the patient to urinate. Meanwhile, froth would come from the mouth and the patient might bite his own tongue.

Great care was necessary to prevent injury or, in extreme cases, death. It was vital to keep a patient in a recovery position, on his side, so that his tongue would not fall back and cause him to choke to death. A mouth gag or a spoon wrapped in a cloth or handkerchief could be inserted above his tongue so that he wouldn't bite his tongue. His clothes had to be loosened to enable him to breathe easier and one had to ensure that the patient fell on something soft and had a cushion for the head to rest on. It was essential that the carer kept the patient under constant observation, to record the length of the convulsion and whether any injury had occurred. Normally a fit or "petit mal" didn't last long and when the patient woke up he might know that he fitted and his medication might have to be reviewed.

Doctors in the psychiatric hospital conducted ECT (electro-convulsive therapy), a recognised treatment for patients suffering from psychosis or schizophrenia, and which caused fitting or convulsion. Mental nurses therefore became experts in caring for epileptics.

One Saturday afternoon we admitted a patient suffering from convulsions every few minutes, an unusual occurrence. He was about thirty years old and had been an epileptic for many years. We were not sure if he had taken his usual medications. In those days we didn't have intensive care and a nurse was designated to observe his fitting, to maintain his airways by using a mouth gag so he wouldn't bite his tongue and to remove his mouth secretions by using a suction machine and a suction catheter.

The patient was almost unconscious and remained fitting for almost three hours, a generalised seizure called a "grand mal". His eyes were rolled up and in the rare moments when he was not fitting, which he was unable to control, he could respond to the nurse's commands. An intravenous infusion was set up to ensure he had an intake of fluids.

The patient could become so exhausted during a "grand mal" that his muscles would tighten and his heart put under so much strain that it could stop and he would die.

It was an unusual and disturbing sight to behold. The patient looked so helpless and frightened and his worried father was by his side. The medical consultant asked for the anaesthetist to assess the patient and it was decided that he had to be rested by putting him to sleep while a ventilator breathed for him. His muscles would relax and in due course he would recover. The medical team would then reintroduce and balance his medication.

This was explained to the patient and he nodded his head. His father agreed and signed the consent form for him. In fact, they had no choice, otherwise he could continue fitting until he died from exhaustion and heart failure. Curare, a poison used at the tip of the arrows of South American Indians to paralyse or kill people or animals, was used to paralyse his body so that a tube could be inserted. The ventilator would then breathe for him and that would give him absolute rest while he was fed intravenously to maintain his life.

His convulsions stopped and the body was rested for two days, during which he was unconscious but washed and cared for. Pressure areas were treated and he was fed well via the intravenous infusion. After two days the consultant gradually re-commenced the anti-epileptic drug via the intravenous infusion. It took three days to balance the drugs and after five days the patient was stable and the doctors decided to wean him off the ventilator.

During the following two days the patient progressed well. He was extubated and was soon able to breathe naturally. He was gradually allowed to eat and drink and on the way to recovery without further convulsion. The medication he received via the infusion was effective and he was subsequently prescribed tablets to be taken orally.

He was a young man and as he began to recover he wouldn't listen to advice and started to complain about the noise on the ward. He convulsed twice during the balancing of his drugs but soon the right balance was found. Unfortunately as he recovered his behaviour became more and more unpleasant. He swore at the doctors and nurses and wanted to go home.

We tried to convince him that he shouldn't go home until

his medication was totally under control but he wouldn't listen. His father was also trying to persuade him to stay but he wouldn't listen to him either. He was becoming louder and louder in his side room and was not at all happy. Eventually the consultant was called but he couldn't convince him to stay so a self-discharge form was signed and he went home twelve days after his admission.

The excellent service provided by the NHS saved this man's life at no cost to him and he angrily discharged himself because he felt we had kept him on the ward unnecessarily. We never heard from him again and were left wondering whether he was alive and well; whether the cause of his epileptic fits was something to do with his behaviour and whether he was taking his medication as prescribed. It was a rare occurrence to see a patient in such an acute phase of epileptic fits and the first-class care of the hospital staff put him well on the road to recovery.

1980s

Tale 19
A Tale of Bad Air

'Respect ghosts and spirits, but keep them at a distance.'
An Eastern saying.

In my charge nurse days I had a good friend who was also Chinese and from Hong Kong. He worked in a psychiatric hospital, his upbringing was similar to mine and we got along very well. Many a time we talked about our lives and times in and around the island of Hong Kong and we could both appreciate what the other was talking about. He told me the following tale about what had happened to his son some months previously. You must decide for yourself whether you believe him, but because of our common background and culture, I certainly do.

Thomas and Philip were both seven years old and very good friends. They had known each other for three years, playing and growing up together. They lived near to one another and played together for most of the time.

There was a recreational park, called "The Rec." at the end of the avenue in which Tom lived and it was a popular place for the youngsters to play. There was a playground at one side, with swings, slides and roundabouts. The middle part was a football pitch where bigger boys tended to play and further down the fields there were woods through which a stream flowed, but not many people went there because it was a bit too far away.

One day Tom and Phil were playing by the edge of the wood and they collected twigs and tried to build a pretend fire. They were doing a good job and had gathered lots of firewood when Tom muttered to himself, "I need a pee."

He went to the side of the wood, took off his jeans and relieved himself on the ground. Suddenly a breeze wafted through the trees and the sky changed colour from grey to yellow and blue. Phil and Tom looked up at the sky, not sure whether they liked what they saw. It was surreal. There was an animal wandering towards them. Tom looked at it and he and Phil retreated to the football pitch where the light seemed brighter and the grass greener.

They continued to play for another twenty minutes, near the swings and slides, and then they went home separately. Tom didn't feel like having his dinner that night. He was looking pale and tired, and later on, in his bedroom, he seemed to wake up and look out of the window. In the morning, he looked unwell and didn't want to eat his breakfast, but his mother cheered him up and sent him off to school. At school he appeared to be half asleep and didn't touch his lunch. After school his mother was informed.

Two days went by and the same thing happened to Tom. Cassie Chan, his mother, was worried and took Tom to see the doctor. On examination, the GP could find nothing wrong and ordered some tests. Tom was looking quite poorly by then. At night, he didn't sleep and stood looking out of the window as if he was hoping to see something. He looked thinner than usual as he had taken only sips of water during the previous few days.

The family doctor was a caring man and dropped by the house to see Tom. He examined him and found no change in his condition. Nothing abnormal was detected and Mrs. Cassie Chan saw the doctor out of the house. Cassie, an attractive English lady, looked worried and tired. A few tears fell from her eyes. She passed by her son's bedroom and offered him a drink of orange juice but Tom sipped a little of it and then shook his head. He looked lethargic and his eyes were sunken.

"I heard what the doctor said," Cassie's husband, James, said. James was in his thirties, good looking and taller than the average Chinese.

"What can we do, James?" Cassie asked anxiously.

The telephone rang.

"Hello. Hello James!"

"Yes. Hello George, what a surprise!" Normally, he would have been more excited.

"Are you ok, brother?" asked George.

"Yes, thanks."

"You don't sound ok at all. Mother was missing you and asked me to ring. She's listening on another line."

"Hello Mum," said James

"Hello James, is anything the matter?"

"Thomas has been feeling poorly for the past few days and hasn't been eating or sleeping well, but the doctor found nothing wrong with him. We're quite worried."

"No temperature?"

"No, Mum."

"Did he eat anything he shouldn't have?" she asked.

"No. He was quite well a few days ago and playing with his friend."

"Perhaps it's nothing to worry about. Ask his friend if they did anything out of the ordinary and we'll ring back in a day or two."

"Thanks Mum, you take care."

"Yes, you too James."

Two days later she rang again.

"Hello James, how's Thomas?"

"No improvement I'm afraid, he could do with a good sleep. He spends most of his time sitting up and looking at something. The doctor has been and suggested he might have to be admitted to hospital soon for a drip feed. Cassie has been crying too. I do wish I knew what's wrong with him."

"I am sorry. Something must have upset him. Did his friend say anything?"

"Only that his friend Phillip said something unusual had happened. They were playing near the woods when a deer appeared as if from nowhere and then disappeared as suddenly as it had appeared."

"Mm......," James' mother was pondering.

"What is it Mum?"

"Leave it with me for a while and I'll try to find out."

"How will you do that? James asked.

"I'll ring you back soon," his mother replied.

"Thanks Mum."

James' mother lived in Wanchai, an overcrowded, residential part of Hong Kong. It was an old, largely unchanged part of the island, little affected by the demands of tourism, its streets congested and the air polluted.

Mrs. Chan was fit for a sixty year old and had no difficulty climbing the steps to the suburban part of Wanchai. She was a kindly woman with greying hair, not tall but quite strong. She entered a building and was greeted by other people as she walked down a long corridor towards the room at the end. Out came an obese woman of similar age. Her face was cheeky and alert.

"Hello, Mrs. Chan," she said.

"Hello, Auntie Mo, I am glad to see you."

"What's the matter, something on your mind?"

"I've brought you some oranges, Mo."

"Thanks, no need for that, but tell me how I can help?"

"My grandson is ill. He can't sleep or eat and my son is very worried."

"Which son is that?" Mo asked.

"It's James, the one living in England."

"Sounds strange, but I'll soon find out."

"Thanks."

"I'll do it now, come inside."

Aunt Mo's room was small and dark. The curtains were drawn and the smell of incense filled the room. In the middle was a statue of a Chinese soldier. His face was red and he had a long black beard, a symbol of righteousness.

Mrs Chan sat down as Mo was lighting more incense in a pot of soil. She also put a small amount of incense in a small bun of her hair, making her appear odd and grotesque. She sat down and mumbled some words, holding a small book of Chinese calendars used for fortune telling. Instantly her face changed from yellow to green and blue, and her voice became high-pitched. It was as if Auntie Mo had gone and was now repossessed.

Mrs. Chan wasn't shocked. She had many years experience

of Chinese culture and had seen this occur before, many years ago, and she believed in its power. The high-pitched voice now turned to that of a man.

"What's the boy's name?"

"Thomas Chan."

"How old is he?"

"Seven."

"Where does he live?"

"In the middle of England."

"Oh!' Auntie Mo's eyes rolled up, her hair stood on end and the incense fell onto the floor. She began to shake as if she was having an epileptic fit and seemed to be in great discomfort.

"Ah, ah, I see an animal, it was a few days ago; a deer. Bad air, bad air! The boy disturbed the bad air."

"What's the bad air?" Chan asked.

"Sorry, sorry," Mo apologised and her voice faded away. She began to be sick and her eyes filled with tears.

"Are you alright, Mo?" Mrs. Chan asked.

Mo woke up gradually and pointed to the tea. Chan brought the tea and her friend took a sip and then sat down properly. She took out a handkerchief, wiped her tears and sipped more tea.

"What did I say, Chan?"

"You saw an animal and the boy disturbed the bad air."

"I thought so."

"What shall I do?"

"Go to the temple."

"Thanks very much, Mo," said Mrs. Chan gratefully, leaving a red pocket of money as a token of gratitude. She then made her way to the Temple.

The Wong Tai Sin temple was a renowned place of worship of the Eastern saints. Many people, young and old, came to worship and have their fortunes told about such things as marriage, business and future prospects. The Temple was renowned for the accuracy of the predictions that were made there.

Mrs. Chan burnt many incense sticks to the Saints of the East and donated money to the Temple. She later talked to a monk who gave her a piece of paper.

The DHL courier service has a reputation for speedy delivery and twenty four hours later a small parcel was delivered to James Chan's home address in Walsall. He read the enclosed note and followed the instructions. He purchased two white triangular paper symbols from a Chinese supermarket in Birmingham and hung them at the top of the window in the doorway of his house. The symbols were called "foofits" and they were blessed in order to keep evil spirits away. Half an hour later his son fell into a deep sleep, snoring away for the first time for many days, and six hours later he woke up and asked for food.

The following day, Chan was guided by his son's friend, Philip, to the recreation field. The boy then headed back home. It was late afternoon, the field was quiet and Chan felt all alone in the world. Fields of oilseed rape glowed a bright yellow colour in the May sunshine. He spread out a picnic of cooked chicken and vegetables, uncorked a bottle of wine and poured two glasses. He then placed two incense sticks in the ground. A chilly breeze sprang up from nowhere but it didn't put out the burning incense. With the wind came the deer, smelling the vegetables and silently approaching the food.

"Please forgive my son," Chan said to the animal.

The animal turned its head and its eyes showed forgiveness. Suddenly the unexpected voice of a little boy came from afar. "Look, it's a deer!"

The animal became angry and pushed Chan to the ground. Chan screamed and took a knife from his back pocket to defend himself, stabbing the deer in the throat. Its blood dripped onto his face and in his fear he could no longer hear his own screaming.

Then he heard a voice crying, "Daddy! Daddy!"

The sound of Thomas' voice woke his father up. Chan looked around at the familiar surroundings of his bedroom. His comely wife was by his side. He looked puzzled.

"Everything is ok, James," she said, placing a tender kiss on his face.

"Is it really?"

"Yes, I went to check if you were alright and I found you lying on the grass. Nothing was left of the picnic and Thomas is now back to his old self. And your mother rang," Cassie continued, "I told her everything is fine. I also told her about Thomas urinating in the field. He couldn't wait any longer. Your mother says he disturbed the peace there and created the bad air."

"Oh yes, I remember when I was small, I was taught to say 'excuse me' if you wanted to disturb the wild."

Thomas came close to his father for a cuddle. "You little devil!" said James Chan, with a smile on his face.

1985

Tale 20
More Unusual Situations

'In life, we all live differently but we all die the same way.'
An Eastern saying.

i) Globus

We all have different problems in our lives, such as work, family, health or educational problems. One of my sons was 18 years old and didn't want to finish his A levels. He was probably the most able of my children, but he wouldn't listen. Instead, he wanted to go off to America to build a computer with an American woman that he met on line. Nothing could persuade him to stay and finish his education,

At work, I had no more than the usual day-to-day problems, nothing that couldn't be solved, but I sensed something at the back of my throat and wondered if I had cancer though I had no difficulty in swallowing. I went to see my family doctor but he was on holiday and I saw a locum who was very young and inexperienced. He examined my throat and ears and could detect nothing abnormal.

I thought of my consultant friend who was an Ear, Nose and Throat specialist. He was always nice to me and agreed to see me very quickly. I explained my problem to him and he agreed to treat me. He passed a narrow tube via my nose into my throat, not a pleasant sensation, and he asked me to look at the television screen which was recording the procedure. It showed some patches of white dots which he said weren't cancer but some kind of throat infection. Antibiotics were prescribed and I took them for two weeks with some success. I went abroad on holiday and felt a little better but I still felt something at the back of my throat. My friend the consultant saw me again and I agreed for him to pass the tube into my throat again to monitor the infection. There were still some dots there but not as many and I was prescribed a further dosage of antibiotics. After five weeks I was much better but still could sense something in my throat. I didn't want to trouble my consultant friend again and made an appointment to see my usual and reliable G.P. who was back from his holidays.

Dr. Pidsley was a middle aged bespectacled man with a professional, friendly manner and I trusted him. I explained my throat problems and he thought a little. "I think I know what's wrong with you, you have globus, but let me take a blood sample for analysis to eliminate other possible illnesses."

"What is globus then?" I asked.

'It's caused by stress and you feel a lump at the back of your throat. I'm quite sure that's what you have and if the blood tests reveal nothing, I shan't contact you and you'll know you have globus," Dr. Pidsley explained.

"How do you treat it then?"

"There's no medication. It won't kill you but you will eventually feel less stressed and the symptoms will disappear."

I went away bemused but remembered the name, "globus".

At home, I looked up globus on the internet and was surprised that there were so many in the world suffering from this complaint. Some people had suffered from it for twenty years. The blood tests were negative, as expected, and soon, the lump in my throat had gone.

A year later, my wife and I went to visit a colleague for dinner. The woman's husband was an orthopaedic surgeon and he told me that he had globus. I had almost forgotten mine, but on reflection, it must have been stress that caused it. I wondered if I still had it or if my body and mind had accepted it as part of my life. Either way, I was quite happy to live with it.

ii) Diagnosis unknown.

One afternoon, a young man was admitted to our medical ward with acute abdominal pain and a high temperature. He was cyanosed, with blue lips and finger tips, and breathless. We gave him oxygen and strong pain killer.

He was about twenty years old and appeared to be very weak and poorly. Several doctors and the consultant on call examined him but their diagnosis was inconclusive. An intravenous infusion was set up for emergency intravenous injections but his heart suddenly stopped beating. The cardiac team arrived and tried unsuccessfully to resuscitate him. The young man's parents looked shocked and helpless and the staff who had tried to save him were devastated.

The following Monday afternoon, a post-mortem had to be performed to find the cause of death and being young and interested I went up to the mortuary with the houseman on call. The body was displayed and opened up. The inside was inspected thoroughly, the brain and heart dissected, but nothing significant was found except a slightly thin chamber of the heart. It was an unpleasant sight, but the mood of the staff was solemn and they wanted to know the cause of death. Unfortunately they were unable to find anything that could explain it.

Why were there situations like this? A life had ended for no reason that medical science could explain. In nursing and medicine, it is a fact of life that there are mysteries that cannot be explained.

One evening in 1988 I was in charge of a surgical ward, and was very busy looking after post-operative surgical patients. In those days, we didn't have day case units dedicated to minor operations and many patients had arrived from the theatre that day.

Mr. Smith was a small man, 78 years old, a patient I had met twice before. He came to the ward every six months to have a routine cystoscopy, a procedure involving the insertion tube via the penis into the bladder to determine whether previously treated tumours had returned. If so, they would be burnt off, using laser treatment.

He returned safely from the operating theatre at 15.00 and at 17.00 he was recovering well. At 18.00, he asked me if he would go home the following day. I replied positively and he went back to his bed, An hour later he was found dead in bed. It was thought he had died of a heart attack.

Many years later, having left the NHS with a fair deal, I was worked in nursing homes for four years. My last nursing home job lasted two years and it was a pleasant learning curve. I looked after older residents and I particularly remember Mrs. Amey, a middle class old lady, well-dressed and very well spoken. I once told her that I was going to Venice for a long weekend and she told me tales about the places she had been, especially the Grand Canal, and the lovely home-made pizzas she had there.

She was 89 years old and had no relatives except a nephew who lived far away. He was her next-of-kin and visited her every six months. Normally, she was jolly and liked me to tell her stories about my career in nursing. We got on very well and because she was very proud of her sewing skills she offered to shorten a pair of trousers for me. She was thrilled when I gave her a big box of chocolates as a thank you.

One day, she told me, "I can't see the point of living and I wish to die."

"Oh no, Mrs. Amey, you can't think like that. We all like you here."

She smiled and two days later went to bed in her room and died peacefully in her sleep. I recall standing at the entrance to her room and saying a prayer for her. God bless you, Mrs. Amey.

iii) Sister Bradley

Sister Mary was a senior sister of a surgical ward. She was an experienced nurse and had been a sister for six years.

"We have a problem, Patrick," she said.

"Oh, what's that?" I asked, trying to stay calm.

"A student told me yesterday that sister Bradley had checked a controlled drug with her and her hand was shaking as if she was having a tremor, and she smelt of alcohol"

"Oh dear, no mistake or drug error I hope?"

"No, thank goodness."

"Ask the nurse to make a statement and we'll take it from there," I said.

"Right."

'Have you noticed anything wrong since you worked with her?" I asked.

"Not really, only that her breath smells sometimes."

"Ok, Mary, we'll see what we can do."

The statement was made and I took it to the senior nursing officer who said it was a difficult situation. Legally, no one can accuse anyone of anything unless they have actually witnessed it.

Later in the day I met Derek, a porter who was also the union representative for NUPE a large union for non-nursing staff. I was quite friendly with him and explained the problem to him without mentioning names. He agreed with the senior nursing officer that unless one actually saw the offence it was not proven.

I discussed the matter with sister Mary and she wasn't happy. We just had to watch sister Bradley and ensure no harm was done. Meanwhile, I talked to her and observed her more closely. She was a stout woman with short brown hair and her dress and demeanour suggested she was not from a well-to-do family. She took my surgical bleep for the evenings and acted as a nursing officer. She always knew what she was doing and made very few mistakes. Tactfully, I asked her if she liked a drink and she said that she did, but never on duty. There was no harm in that, I thought; perhaps that was the reason she sometimes smelt of drink.

Two weeks went by and sister Mary advised me that another suspicious situation had arisen at 15.30, giving me an opportunity to watch sister Bradley that evening. I went purposely and did a spot check on the entire controlled drug store, which was one of my duties. Controlled drugs were addictive drugs and their storage and use was governed by the Controlled Drug Act. All controlled drugs administered had to be checked by a qualified nurse and another person, and all had to be signed for. These drugs included morphine and pethidine both of which had a very high value on the black market.

I checked the drugs with sister Bradley, who was rather nervous, and found them all correct.

"Are you feeling alright, sister?" I asked.

"Not bad, but I didn't sleep well last night."

"Oh, is there anything you want to tell me?"

"Like what?" She asked.

I shrugged my shoulders and said nothing.

"Is there anything you want to tell me, Patrick?"

"Well, actually there is" I said, trying to be as tactful as I could. "Some nurses on the ward say that sometimes your hands shake when you check the drugs with them, and that you smell of alcohol as if you have been drinking."

"Oh, is that all? I have recently changed my perfume which smells like alcohol."

"Perhaps you ought to change it to avoid confusion."

"Perhaps, but I can't see why I should. I like the perfume."

"Well, I can't insist, but if you do have a drink problem you should go to the staff health department."

"Ok, I'll bear that in mind, but I really don't have a problem, you know."

At least, she now knew that we were all watching her.

Sister Bradley never went to occupational health for help and these suspicions hung around the surgical unit for two years. Nothing was ever proven and Sister Bradley went on to become a district sister. It was one of many unusual incidents in my career.

Three years went by and I was promoted to another job in a nearby town. At a nursing conference, I met one of the surgical sisters I worked with in my previous job and we started talking about old times. "Do you remember Sister Bradley?" she asked.

"How can I forget?"

"She killed herself last week with a shotgun in her garage."

"Oh dear, that's awful." I was shocked.

"And it was said that she had been drinking."

"Really?"

I wished that Sister Bradley had taken my advice to seek help, but perhaps that was too simple a solution.

Tale 21
Andy's Deception

'Into the wind shall lightly pass the pain.' Nicholas Grimald.

It was a typically busy Friday afternoon with endless emergency admissions on the surgical ward. We had admitted six patients ranging from abdominal pains to acute appendicitis. Abdominal pains were a common cause of admissions on the ward and the causes varied so much, including severe constipation, obstructions and tumours.

The ward telephone rang. We were told that we were going to admit a patient with renal colic, causing haematuria, meaning the presence of blood in the urine. Andy was the patient's name. He was very pale and rolling in bed with a colicky pain. He told us that the oral analgesic hadn't helped and that the doctor had prescribed an injection of pethidine, a controlled drug for severe pain. I checked with another nurse and gave Andy the injection, which was effective almost immediately, and he thanked us for helping to relieve the pain. He was thin and in his late twenties, unusually young to have renal stones causing the colicky pain.

A student nurse was on duty and kept asking me

questions. I explained that renal colic was a common reason for admission to an acute surgical ward and that it was mostly due to kidney stones blocking a renal blood vessel. Andy's pain was quite characteristic as patients usually rolled about in bed with a severe spasmodic pain on the kidney side. Andy was advised to pass his urine in a bottle so that we could test it for blood. We also wanted to observe whether he passed any stones by sieving his urine. The first sample did indicate some traces of blood in his urine. The test was done by the use of a labstix. The labstix was dipped in the urine and the change of the colour indicated the presence of blood. The urine was sieved and there were no stones found. The student nurse was quite intrigued by it all.

During the night, Andy had pethidine every six hours according to the doctor's orders and it helped. Before the injection, he was in pain, with tremors, shaking vigorously and looking pale. The staff thought he was very unlucky and so young to have such a complaint, because patients were usually older, obese and had a high cholesterol level. Andy could not always urinate to provide a specimen when we asked. In fact, we obtained only one specimen from him. However, when we asked again on Saturday he did produce some urine. I looked at it with the houseman called Mick.

"That's blood, isn't it?" he said.

I nodded my head in agreement and we looked at each other and smiled.

Mick was a young doctor, about 28 years old, efficient and quite shrewd. He was obviously thinking what I was thinking. He prescribed a sterile water injection instead of pethidine. It could be viewed as unethical to prescribe an injection of sterile water in lieu of a pain killer, but the method worked because when the next injection was due Andy showed signs of distress. He asked for the pain killer but the injection of sterile water was given again and it worked as effectively as the analgesic. Mick and I smiled wryly and we both thought that he might have cut himself to mix the blood in his urine.

Our suspicion grew and I looked at the folder of regional health warnings. These were circulars we received regularly that advised us to be on the lookout for dubious characters. One of them advised us that there was a young man who had been admitted to several hospitals asking for pethidine and feigning to be suffering from severe pain. The description of the young man fitted Andy.

Pethidine was a controlled drug, made from heroin, that was used treat severe pain but it was addictive and some drug addicts became addicted to it. I went to Andy's bed and asked further questions about his life history. He told me that he was visiting his aunt who lived in the town and that he normally lived in a city a hundred miles away. I could see that he was feeling uncomfortable with my questioning. He was waiting for a scan on his kidneys on Monday, and by Sunday he had been given two placebo pain killers that seemed to have been effective, but he was now asking for a stronger painkiller. Mick was talking to him about this and he asked Andy if he was addicted to any drugs. Andy became agitated and angry.

"What do you mean, Doc? Are you accusing me of being a drug addict?"

"No. It's just a routine question. Why are you so angry?" asked Mick.

Andy didn't answer.

I showed him the circular about a young man in the West Midlands, feigning suffering and asking for strong pain killers.

In the black market, an ampoule of pethidine would be worth a lot of money. Andy was now losing his temper and accusing us of being unprofessional and uncaring. He packed his bag and stormed out of the ward. I told him that it was his right to discharge himself and if he would sign the self-discharge form he could go. He scribbled his signature and quickly left the ward.

In most NHS general hospitals, many emergency admissions occurred during the weekends, some of them might be routine overdose patients, taking paracetamol and aspirin, and some seemed to enjoy the stomach washouts. Some swallowed knifes or forks which showed up on X-rays and the staff knew these people well. We also had our regular drunks who would disturb the ill patients on the wards. They woke up, urinated on the beds and discharged themselves the following morning, not waiting to be seen by senior doctors. The purpose of this kind of behaviour might have been to draw attention to themselves. In addition to our regular customers we had patients like Andy, wandering through NHS hospitals and obtaining free injections of strong pain killers.

In some university towns, militant students believed in extreme utopian ideas and the admission of students suffering from overdoses were common at weekends. Indeed, the staff in the hospitals, the doctors, nurses and porters, would sometimes be subjected to abuse, and even physical violence from the so-called patients.

All these services were free of charge from the NHS.

1982

Tale 22
The Worst Jobs in Nursing

'Somebody has to do it ...'

When I was a senior nurse in a surgical unit I was involved in teaching and assessing student nurses and the local College of Nursing often asked me to give guest lectures on development courses for trained nurses. These courses aimed to equip them with the knowledge and skills necessary to teach and assess other nurses. I was also asked to take the chair at seminars for students and trained nurses and at one seminar the question arose as to what jobs were considered to be the worst in nursing.

At the top of the list was the inspection of sputum samples. This seemed to be most off-putting for many nurses, especially female nurses, yet all nurses were well trained in the science and art of observation. The observation by doctors and nurses of the contents of sputum pots was a vital part of the job. I knew it well, as I had been a charge nurse on a medical ward for some three years.

We were trained to observe, for instance, whether the sputum was frothy, infected, and whether it was green or yellow in colour. A keen observer could rapidly obtain information about the general state of the patient from the colour, consistency and amount of sputum. For instance, frothy green sputum could infer an acute infection by a strain of haemolytic streptococci and invariably, after analysis by the pathology laboratory, the diagnosis was confirmed. Yellowish sputum could indicate whether the patient was suffering from a chest infection or whether the correct antibiotics had been used, and if the patient had coughed-up lots of sputum it might mean the patient's chest was loosening-up. Blood in the sputum (haemoptysis) could indicate cancer of the airway, lungs, or tuberculosis.

This was empirical science at its best, the collection and observation of sputum being a very important procedure, capable of identifying the cause of an illness or disease, which in turn could indicate the appropriate course of treatment.

The next unsavoury task was the observation of vomit. Vomit was unpleasant to observe, collect and to clear up, but the sample could provide a clear clinical diagnosis of the patient's illness, and the prognosis. I remember a patient in a nursing home bringing up some brown-coloured vomit and the trained nurse disposed of it, but a care assistant collected another specimen and showed it to me. I thought that, with the other symptom of constipation, the patient might be suffering from an intestinal obstruction. The GP was called and he agreed with me, sending the patient urgently to hospital where an intestinal obstruction was confirmed and unblocked by the surgeon just in time. The GP congratulated me on the observation and I praised the care assistant for his good work.

Brown-coloured vomit could also indicate some form of

haemorrhage in the lower alimentary tract, lower intestinal obstruction or trauma. If, however, the vomit contained bright coloured or fresh blood, it would be indicative of problems in the upper alimentary tract; for instance, ulcers, tumours, acute infection or poisoning. Hence, the observation of vomit was a very important part of nursing care.

No one likes the look of faeces but all doctors and nurses have to observe and learn about them. Blood in a stool could indicate constipation or cancer of the bowel and a black stool might indicate a side effect of taking iron tablets or bleeding from the upper intestinal tract. The high frequency of passing a stool might be indicative of ulcerative colitis. In the world of nursing, many old-fashioned ward sisters saw themselves as experts in helping patients to 'open their bowels' by using senokots, lactulose syrup, suppositories, enemas or washouts. Many nurses took pride in the belief that they had more expertise in that department than doctors! Extreme constipation, e.g. not going to the toilet for five or six days, or constant diarrhoea, could be a symptom of cancer of the bowel. The odour emitting from the stool is also of interest. For example, an extremely offensive smell could indicate a lack of bile salts, natural chemicals produced by the liver to deodorise the faeces. Absence of these bile salts often preceded obstructive jaundice or other serious hepatic disorders.

The observation of urine is another vital skill required of all nurses and doctors. The frequency of passing, its colour, content and amount might all indicate symptoms of diseases. Dribbling of urine is common in older men because of an enlarged prostate gland. Blood in the urine (haematuria) might indicate stones in the kidneys or cancer of the bladder.

Painless haematuria is usually a bad sign that could indicate cancer of the bladder or kidney and, because it is painless, it is often ignored. The colour of the urine is an important indication as to whether a patient is drinking enough. Clear urine of a light amber colour indicates a sufficient intake of liquids whereas dark coloured urine could indicate not drinking enough. This is often associated with pain in the bladder, indicating urinary tract infection, which is one of the most common disorders in the elderly.

There were occasions when nurses asked me to describe the most unusual thing I had seen. It was an enormous scrotal hernia, perhaps just slightly larger than a baby's head, and we had to raise the foot of the bed to try to reduce it. The patient was in real danger of the hernia blocking part of his intestine and the poor man was on bed rest for several days before his operation. After the operation the hernia remained, but a little smaller and he was eventually discharged with a huge scrotal support. The nurses relished their discussions at the seminars and the students learnt quite a lot. Many confessed that their worst experience was seeing or changing their first colostomy bag, first leg amputation or burst abdomen. Needless to say, the discussion would often develop into something even more off-putting, such as what caused our first fainting in nursing.

I confessed that the only time I felt light-headed and needed to sit down was at my first experience of electro-convulsive-therapy in a mental hospital. I was helping the doctors to administer the procedure for patients suffering from psychosis or schizophrenia and in 1968 we seldom used pre-medications like Scolin injections to relax patients before ECT. As in the movie "One Flew Over the Cookoo's Nest" they administered all the ECT "in the raw." I was one of six men helping the patient, who would have had neither food nor drink for six hours, and he would have a wedge to bite on so that he wouldn't bite his tongue. Our job was to apply compression to the shoulders, hips and feet so the patient wouldn't jerk and dislocate his joints. I was asked to press on one of his hips.

When the doctor connected the wire to the patient's head and put on the switch, the patient would receive an electric shock. He would shake and jerk and an epileptic fit would be induced for a few minutes. The violent spasms of were a shocking sight to behold with the patients frothing at the mouth. Once the seizure subsided, the patient would relax and turn from rigid to relaxed, quite often urinating in his trousers. He would then be carried from the stretcher and transferred to a mattress in the dormitory. We often dealt with up to ten patients in a morning.

This treatment looked barbaric and after two procedures I felt slightly faint. I was a teenager at the time and I can recall it as if it were only yesterday. ECT was effective in the treatment of psychosis and schizophrenia but was never scientifically proven. It is still in use today but is often helped by the use of injections to relax the patients before being applied.

The students were intrigued by these stories and often started to confess their worst experiences. The commonest examples were witnessing their first post mortem, helping in the operating theatre for the first time or watching an awkward dressing. Fainting was not uncommon when witnessing something like this for the first time, but it didn't put us off our chosen vocation.

1990

Tale 23
Chan's dream

'Tread softly because you tread on my dreams.' W.B. Yeats.

In Tale 19 I wrote about my old friend and male nurse, Chan, and his supernatural tale. I believed it because like most Chinese, I am superstitious. He also told me once about how a dream helped his brother to shape his son's future.

Chan was a hard working driver in Hong Kong. He was not really old, only thirty-five years of age, but the driving world in the seventies was a man's world and Chan never had the opportunity to meet many girls. He eventually succumbed to the old Chinese method of finding a woman; an arranged date.

He looked at many photographs, chose a woman and met her in a Chinese restaurant. He liked her because she was quite attractive and had a strong personality. She had experienced the tougher world of Old China and had worked hard in a factory in Hong Kong. Their courtship wasn't a long one and after a few months, they were married. Chan had a meek and easy-going manner. His family was too poor to send him to school, so they borrowed money so that he could learn to drive and eventually he made a living by driving.

Chan soon had a son whom he loved but one day his son had a high temperature and his wife wanted to delay taking him to see a doctor because it would cost more money than they could afford. Unfortunately the wait proved to be fatal. Their son convulsed and was admitted to hospital as an emergency where he soon died of a high temperature. The Chans were devastated, especially Chan himself. He drank and cried and felt so sad and lost for a long time. His wife was tougher and tried to console him. "We will make another baby, do not worry, husband." She was clearly the stronger one in the partnership.

Soon she became pregnant again and they had another son, Trevor. Chan was so happy but he never forgot his first son. At times, he dreamt of him and he told him how much he missed him. As time went on, Chan became preoccupied with his second son, but he was frequently unwell during the first 18 months of his life. He was weak and prone to infections. Many of the parents' relatives commented on this and Chan and his wife were worried. They bought the best food for him to eat and looked after him very well but Trevor remained lethargic and weak.

One night, Chan dreamt of his first son again, the first time for a long time. His son asked, "Dad, why are you not happy?"

"Your brother is not well and we don't want to lose him as we lost you. Are you well, son.?"

"No, dad. Perhaps that is why Trevor is always poorly."

"Why do you say this? We loved you and we regretted not taking you to the doctor sooner."

"It isn't your fault, Dad."

"Tell me son, what I should do?"

The dream ended abruptly, with his son crying. Chan thought his son was sad. He felt he was drowning and woke up in a sweat, from a nightmare.

"What is the matter?" his wife asked.

"Just a nightmare. I dreamt of our first son, the first time for a long time."

"Don't be silly."

"I used to dream about him a lot."

"Go back to sleep."

Chan had a similar dream about his dead son again and again and sensed that he was not at peace. He thought of visiting his grave for the first time since the funeral ceremony. He hadn't visited the grave because he knew he would feel so sad afterwards, but this time he knew he had to visit it. It was no good asking his wife to accompany him as she was tougher than him.

When he visited the grave he could not believe what he saw. It was surrounded by water, with little drainage around the gravestone. Weeds had overgrown the grave and it looked neglected and uncared for. Chan instructed a grave digger to tidy-up the site, remove all the weeds and dig a channel for the water to drain away. When this was done the grave looked more presentable and at peace. He burnt incense, whispered words of peace to his son, and then Chan sobbed and cried uncontrollably. He stood there for a long time and the passers-by felt sorry for him. A chill wind came from nowhere, cooling Chan down, and suddenly, he stopped crying. A feeling of ease enveloped him. Feeling better, he bowed his head three times in front of the grave and said a fond farewell to his first son.

I'm sorry I didn't come to see you more often, please forgive me as I got so upset when I was here, but I will come every year at Ching Ming time. The Ching Ming festival was the time the Chinese paid their respects to the dead.

That night Chan's dead son came to him in a dream once more.

"Hello son," Chan said.

"Dad, please don't get so upset over me, I am dead and gone."

"Yes, but are you alright?"

"I am now, since you tidied up my grave."

"I'm so sorry I neglected it."

"Don't blame yourself, you will be a wonderful father to Trevor and he will be fine now. I have made a blessing for him and he will be a good and successful son to you."

"Really?"

"Yes, goodbye Dad, I cannot talk to you again, I am at peace."

"But I will miss you so much."

"I know you will. Take care of yourself, Dad."

Chan went to sleep peacefully and woke up feeling well and comfortable.

From then on, Trevor Chan had a healthy life. He was hard working and studied diligently. Twenty-five years later he became a chartered accountant and the co-owner of a Japanese restaurant and, true to his word, Chan visited his son's grave every year during the Ching Ming festival.

Tale 24
The NHS & Community Care Act 1990

'Her plot hath many changes: every day speaks a new scene.'
F.Quarles

Over the past twenty years or so there has been much in the newspapers about hospitals being in the red and staff, including doctors, nurses and support staff, being made redundant. Cuts have made everywhere in the NHS and one wonders what brought it all about. It was a common topic of conversation and debate amongst my tennis-playing friends in the 1980s, when Margaret Thatcher was in power. In 1988 she announced a root and branch review of the NHS. A White Paper was published the following year and it became law as the NHS & Community Care Act 1990.

I was an operational manager at Burton hospital at the time and we were well advanced with computerisation. A group of managers was invited to Kings Fund Hospital, London, to receive training on resource management. The concept was unique and we were one of the pilot schemes for the computerisation of most of the activities in the hospital. In addition, the management structure was to be totally changed.

I was studying for the Diploma in Health Service Management at the time and had learnt much about the proposed changes. Our lecturer used to say jokingly, "In the old days, hospitals were managed by an administrator and his dog, with a little help from a senior consultant and the top nurse." In future, hospitals would be divided into many different specialties, such as surgery, medicine, children's services and so on. In each specialty there would be a senior nurse, a senior consultant, a business manager, and attached to the unit would be an accountant. This was called a Resource Management Directorate. All activities would be discussed in this directorate and buying and selling services would be developed. Everything would be looked at carefully in terms of cost and quality to determine whether or not we could afford it.

Some consultants questioned where the money would come from to fund these business managers and accountants, and the reply was, from existing budgets. In short, funding these new posts would decrease the budgets of the medical specialties. We had no choice but to implement the new structure. It was an order from above and the government believed that once the structure was in place hospitals would save money.

The senior management structure was bringing in amazing changes which were beneficial to some managers. Before the changes, we had administrators but their titles were changed to directors and we had directors of estates, finance, hospitality services and so on, all much more highly paid than their previous jobs. They did have more responsibility but their salaries were increased out of all proportion. All aspects of the hospital were looked at in terms of cost and, if we could afford it, quality. There were no increases in budgets; savings were made from clinical services. No wonder the unions protested but their protests were to no avail.

The concept of purchasing and selling was introduced. Hospitals like ours would be the providers and we would sell our services to purchasers who would buy them or not, depending on price and quality. Endless meetings were set up to discuss these purchasing and providing services. One of the implications was that patients might have to travel many miles for the best care and there were debates as to whether a patient would travel fifty miles for an operation that was previously available on the doorstep. Some might and some might not. In practice, there were other implications, such as whether relatives and other visitors would travel fifty miles to visit a sick patient.

All senior managers would be on performance related pay (PRP) and the top manager had to keep control of the budget, never mind the other important issues. Bonuses would be awarded if budgets were met. Never before had we ever looked at costs and budgets in this way.

All these changes had devastating effects on the wards. Hospitals decided that they couldn't afford to employ cooks to prepare meals on site because it was cheaper to have them centrally cooked five weeks in advance and frozen or chilled until they were required. Patients were assured that the nutritional value would be the same. Hospital canteen staff wouldn't eat the food, but the patients had no choice! It was claimed that the system would be cheaper.

The ward sisters were the kingpins of the wards as they were in control of all activities, including domestic, hygiene and cleaning functions, but following the decentralisation domestics were employed by a company many miles away and the ward sisters couldn't alter their practices. They had to complain to managers of firms miles away. I wondered if this change in accountability was the cause of the significant increase in ward infections.

From newspaper reports and other media research I was able to confirm the sharp increase in the number of managers in hospitals. The NHS & Community Care Act went further and changed GPs (general practitioners) into fund holders, employing practice managers to oversee the operation of surgeries. Their main focus was on income and expenditure.

This drastic change in the operation of the NHS had a tremendous impact on the services provided and when the Tory government was eventually replaced by New Labour it was too late, too costly and too disruptive to turn back the clock. The new NHS structure and practices were kept in place and the service continued to deteriorate. The directors became more powerful and more highly paid. Chief executives were paid more than £100,000 a year and on the wards the staff were paid proportionately less for doing more work. Morale was sinking lower and lower.

Last week, September, 2012, I was reading a newspaper and learnt that medical consultants had to dictate their reports for transmission to India where they would be typed by local women on much lower wages than British women. Gone were the days when medical secretaries worked closely with consultants, when secretaries would be familiar with patients' medical histories and would listen to their concerns and complaints.

If the concept and purpose of the trusts, directorates and the internal market was effective, one might ask why many of them have gone bust. Is it because the managers were inefficient, the funds allocated wrongly, that managers were paid more at the expense of the clinical work?

The NHS & Community Care Act created a group of people destined to be winners. They were the "yes men," people with a talent for talking. They agreed with everything and didn't ask for reasons. Such was the integrity of these people that I knew of one man who, in order to survive, would not only give a sweet to the boss to sugar him up, he actually unwrapped the sweet for the boss and almost put it in his mouth! He soon became a director and wore silk ties and made-to-measure suits. Soon, the NHS was full of such people. They were whiz kids with eloquent tongues, always ready to say what bosses liked to hear in order to get a senior job. They would change the systems and procedures that had worked well for decades and after a year or two they were off to seek further promotion. It was a sad fact that many good employees, men and women with integrity, commitment and a sense of vocation failed to survive the upheaval.

In my view, the NHS Community Care Act 1990 resulted in major changes which have caused significant damage to the health of patients, yet, by many it is regarded as a success and now the same ideology is spreading into education.

1994

Tale 25
Stress in the National Health Service

'You can't get a quart into a pint pot.' British proverb.

It is common knowledge that in the National Health Service there is a major reorganisation every two or three years. During the latter part of my career in the NHS many employees, especially amongst the senior staff, felt they had no security, although if they had been in the NHS for more than three years and had to change jobs their salaries were protected for five years.

A glut of White Papers seemed to suggest that new ways were always better than the old, but no one had bothered to count the cost of the numerous reorganizations which had become a way of life in the NHS.

Of all my nursing staff, Sister Skit was probably the most popular and respected. She was well-liked by patients, doctors and nurses, and I never heard anyone speak badly of her. She was caring, patient, polite, and had the best bedside manner anyone had ever seen. Change seemed to be a way of life to her. She took all changes and upheavals in her stride.

She was the manager of the Ear, Nose and Throat ward,

a skilled area of specialty nursing. She was always composed and in control, and during the eight years I had known her, I had never seen her lose her temper. On many occasions I left my bleep with her to stand in for me on the surgical unit and she never complained. I was sad when I heard that she was retiring and wondered who could take over from her and match her composure and professionalism. At her retirement party I praised her kindness, commitment and dedication to her work, and because she didn't drive I offered to give her a lift home afterwards.

"Well, Ann, I'm going to miss you. It was a good party, wasn't it?" I said as I drove her home.

"Yes, very nice indeed, thank you for organising it for me," she replied. "You always said that you wanted to do some other kind of work didn't you Patrick?"

"Yes, but I don't know what. I suppose I've only known working in the NHS, a very sheltered life."

"But it is secure."

"Yes, I suppose it is, and fairly well-paid too."

"At least I can sleep well now," said Ann, sounding relieved.

"But you are always so relaxed, I thought you always slept well."

"No! I haven't slept well for 10 years. These continuous changes in responsibilities can be a very great burden to a ward manager."

"But you always appeared to be composed and in control."

"I suppose I'm a great pretender, but I do worry and have never slept well."

"Now you tell me, on your last day. You've really shocked me."

"Well, you can't get a quart of fluid into a pint pot, you know."

"But you never let it get you down. You always stood tall and upright, Ann!"

"Have you heard about Albert, the deputy unit general manager?" asked Ann, abruptly changing the subject.

"I did hear that he's ill," I replied.

"I'm afraid it's more than that."

"Oh, what is it then, I've heard very little?"

"He lives quite near to me and I've noticed he looks very drawn and anxious."

"I'm sorry to hear that. I've always found the UGM to be a quiet, pleasant man; very conscientious and hard working, but I haven't seen him for a while. There again, I don't meet the senior managers very often. Tell me more."

"Well, I've heard his wife is not very nice and she's going to leave him."

"Oh dear!" I was shocked. Albert was only in his thirties and had a young daughter.

"Apparently he was under a lot of pressure from work and was found wandering around Birmingham. He didn't know his own name."

"Bloody hell!" I exclaimed. "All this stress can manifest itself in different ways and you have to be very strong to survive. I'm really sorry for him."

"The whole village felt for him," said Ann.

'"I must inquire further about him," I said, as I dropped Ann off at her house. She got out of the car, I gave her a kiss on the cheek and thanked her for all the work she had done for the unit. She smiled and we wished each other all the best.

On the way home, rain was falling and the sky was grey. Sister Ann had coped very well with the stress throughout her nursing career. It was one of the biggest killers in the NHS.

Shortage of staff, increased workloads and endless change ground one down. As for poor Albert, I heard later that his wife had left him with their daughter and he never came back to work.

On reflection, there were indeed many episodes of duty from which I went home worried about the ward's staff situation and the workload. The wards were often under-staffed and requests for help to my colleague nursing officers fell on deaf ears. The Director was contacted but it seemed every ward was in the same situation, either under-staffed or working with the bare minimum. No wonder Sister Skit couldn't sleep well. The situation was the same in my previous job as the middle line manager for surgical areas. Very often the wards were operating with just a skeleton staff.

Once, when I was a charge nurse, after a very busy day on the wards, with endless information coming in from consultants and doctors, I woke up at two in the morning and rang the night sister to give her some information that I had forgotten to tell her before I went off duty. The stress must have been there all the time, but we ward sisters never spoke about it. We were reluctant to complain because it might be taken as an indication that we were not managing our work as well as we should. We just bottled it up, soldiered on and did the best we could.

1987

Tale 26
A Major Disaster

'A winning team is greater than the sum of its parts.'

After a reorganisation I was appointed to the post of operational manager of the surgical unit, in charge of nurses and non-nurses, a total of 120 staff. I was a little nervous about it because it was the first time I had been responsible for units or specialties I didn't know much about, such as orthodontics and audiology. I assumed that because I had passed my diploma in health service management, the senior staff thought I knew enough to do the job.

I relished the challenge and found the staff interesting. They were the heads of the dental laboratory, audiological department and medical secretaries. All were as nervous as I was in our first meeting but we had to make it work and as time went on, we understood each other better and worked very well together.

Our manager's boss was very proactive man. He was a part-time Territorial Army NCO and relished it. He decided that all managers on our grade needed some leadership training and booked us on an outward bound course. A group of us, all middle managers, were sent for a long residential weekend at a Shropshire cottage where we were put through a series of progressively more challenging exercises. We were a bit weary after the abseiling and walking on a narrow rope across a lake but Bert, the senior head, emphasised that health and safety was of paramount importance to all of us.

Food and lodging was provided and we regarded the days spent on the course as work days. I met many heads of department I never met before; heads of X-ray, physiotherapy and catering, to name a few. A hospital was a huge place and although some people were familiar to me, having met them in the hospital corridors, I didn't really know them. The event was successful in bringing us together as a team and it was also enjoyable, light-hearted and fun.

We all walked successfully across the lake on the narrow rope, all of us looking straight ahead and treading carefully. I didn't like heights but managed to complete the only abseil of my life. Clues were hidden in the countryside and we had to work through the night as teams to find them. We built a raft and paddled out onto the lake to recover an object. It was great fun and we all thoroughly enjoyed the event, in spite of the lack of sleep. Having never done anything like it before, I found it memorable and, in terms of management training, very effective. I was rather sad to say goodbye to some of the heads of department because, once back at work in the hospital, we were unlikely to meet, and if we did we would be in a rush to complete some task or other.

One Saturday, two months later, I was on call when we received an emergency call for a major disaster. Major disasters were rare in our small town, in spite of the fact that we were near to the A38 trunk road. Two vans had collided and some fourteen people were injured, two of them seriously. We didn't know until later that all of them were Indians, and all bearing the surname Patel.

Mr. Selwyn was the surgical consultant and we knew and worked well with each other. I called in various staff, as per procedure for a major disaster, and they were very willing to turn out because a major disaster was so rare. Fortunately, there were a few empty beds available and some consultants co-operated by discharging patients early to allow new admissions. Many heads of department came in, as required for a major disaster, and it was pleasing to meet some I had met on the outward bound training weekend. We all pulled together as a team for the good of the patients, all of whom were cared for well, but we had to be careful with their names as they were all called Patel.

Two patients needed operations and they were soon on the way to recovery. The nurses were all so co-operative and helped each other in any way they could. It was a pleasure to see. The other patients had all sustained various kinds of fractures and the outpatients and orthopaedic units were extremely busy. Those of us who were involved in the outward bound training reflected how effective the training had been in enabling us to work so effectively as a team. In the small hours of the morning we all felt very tired but happy and satisfied that we had done a good job.

A few days later, I was called upon to be part of a team, together with a senior hospital manager, to conduct an audit of the event. It was a fairly lengthy process but we learnt from the incident that we must establish a temporary unit number for each patient because it was confusing having so many patients with the same surname. Overall, we were praised for having coped well and many of us felt that the outward bound training had made a valuable contribution to the successful handling of this major disaster.

1993

Tale 27
Albert and Lisa

'Each time you fall down, just get back up and move on.'
Soka Gakkai.

During my last year at Newmarket, when I was working to complete my training, many more Chinese students arrived. Word must have travelled around Hong Kong and suddenly we had some thirty pupil nurses in training, mostly women. We had been the treasured few, but no longer. It seemed Chinese students were everywhere in the hospital, probably because it was difficult to find local people to train as nurses, and very soon problems started to occur. Some Chinese students were not as polite as they should have been, and spoke Cantonese everywhere, even in front of the English staff. I thought such behaviour was rude and inexcusable, and that didn't make me the most popular person in the hospital. Additionally, some Chinese girls dated English doctors and amorous tales began to circulate.

Albert, my Chinese pupil colleague, lived near to me in the male nurses' home. We started in the same group and we were progressing well. He appears to have been chased by a

Chinese girl, Lisa, and Albert liked her too. Lisa gradually took over the care of Albert's room, acting as unofficial, unpaid housekeeper. She kept things very tidy, sometimes cooked for him and became quite possessive. I seldom saw Albert after he met Lisa and wondered whether she wouldn't allow him to see me. I was naïve and silly and commented to Albert one day that it seemed abnormal that Lisa had taken over his life. He must have repeated this to Lisa and from then on she avoided me. In fact, when we finished our training at Newmarket, Albert went on to continue his training elsewhere and we didn't see each other for another twenty years.

My wife came from Wellingborough, a small town in Northamptonshire, and we visited her parents once or twice a year. One Saturday I was wandering in the town by myself. There were many people about and suddenly I saw a grey haired man with a familiar face and I knew I had met him before. He nodded to me as if he knew me as well.

"Hey, Albert!" I said.

"Patrick! We haven't met for more than twenty years."

"Long time no see, Albert," I said, as we shook hands, "I'm very pleased to see you again after so many years. Do you live in Wellingborough.?"

"Yes, very near here, in a flat; and what you doing here?"

"Visiting the in-laws; they have been living here for many years."

"Really? I've been living here for five years. Would you like to come round for a cup of tea in my place?"

"Yes, sure." I knew we had twenty years to catch up with.

His flat was small but immaculately tidy. We recounted our times in Newmarket where we spent two and a half years together, working as a pupil nurse. Now we were both trained and registered general nurses. I was a senior nurse in surgery and he was just leaving his job as a charge nurse to work as a senior nurse in a Health Authority in Lincolnshire.

He told me the story of his life since we parted in Newmarket. Lisa was in love with him and they both left Newmarket to be trained as registered nurses in Hertfordshire where they were later married. They were very happy together and soon Lisa became pregnant with twin boys. Over the years Lisa became progressively more possessive and followed Albert around wherever he went. After the twins were born, he found a second job as an agency nurse, in addition to his job as a staff nurse in the local hospital. His two salaries enabled the family to live in comparative comfort in their lovely detached four bedroom house. I told him that I had married an English girl, that we had four children and we were living happily in Burton Upon Trent.

One day, Albert returned from work and found all the door locks had been changed and he couldn't get in. He was panicking and telephoned Lisa.

"Why can't I get in the house?" he asked.

"Well, Albert, I've had enough. I wasn't born to raise your twin boys. It's too much for me and I want to keep the house and you can leave with the boys."

Her words were like knife plunging into Albert's heart. "You can't do that, it's my house as well," he protested.

They quarrelled bitterly for a while before Albert moved back into the house but it was obvious it wouldn't work and eventually he moved out with the boys. He bought himself a flat in Wellingborough and was soon promoted to charge nurse. Life was tough for him, raising the twins himself, and shortly afterwards Lisa and he were divorced. I found it difficult to believe that a wife and mother could behave in such a way, not wanting to know or to raise her own sons.

Albert was resilient and disciplined. He had the grit and determination to work hard, and succeeded in raising the twins very well. They both went to university while Albert himself completed an MBA. He was very careful with money but the family lived a comfortable life.

When we parted that afternoon I still found it difficult to believe his story and we met once a year for the following few years. Lisa, having heard the twins were doing well, contacted Albert, and wanted to come back after all the years of neglecting them. She sent them birthday cards but the twins and Albert ignored them and didn't want to see her again. I felt very sorry for Albert as he had no woman friends, although he told me that several times after the divorce women had tried to get close to him, but he was cautious and apprehensive about entering another relationship and he never had a serious girlfriend again.

Years later, we both retired from the NHS with a good pension and we met yearly to reflect on what we had achieved. We didn't have any communication from our former peers in Newmarket but we heard that some of them had gone back to Hong Kong and others to Australia. Albert's sons did very well and made lots of money in the banking world. Albert became a Justice of Peace and I became an External Verifier for an Awarding Body.

Albert was the first man that I befriended when I came to England and now we are both much older, more grey, and hopefully wiser, we relish our companionship more. His sons have done better than mine financially but I don't mind that as it was beyond my control. Both of us have done rather well in our lives and we are both quite reconciled with the world.
1993

Tale 28
Nurses' Pay

'The love of money is the root of all evil.'
First epistle of Paul to the Thessalonians.

Since I joined the nursing profession in England in 1969 I have been an avid reader of the Nursing Times, the leading professional nursing journal in this country. The journal has a long history in England and also has an international circulation. Over the years I have made two or three contributions, including the following, on nurses' pay, published on March 13th 1991.

Dear Editor,
PRB Fails Senior Managers
I am afraid I don't share the views of your editorial (February 12th) on the Pay Review Body. The PRB has done a bad job as far as I am concerned, and I'm sure that thousands of nurses of senior grade 6 and above would agree. Because we are in a minority, (only 2000 to 3000 in the country) we have not succeeded in the pay negotiations and have been bullied by the government. The PRB has achieved very little for us.

I work as a nurse manager, as do my grade I colleagues, and I am also the assistant to a director of nursing services. I have specific responsibility for manpower, computer work and, in the frequent absence of my boss, am responsible for many grade I and H nurses. I used to be a grade 5, while my colleagues were grades 7 or 8, but they are now all grade I and H, and earning far more than I do.

I know I am not the only senior nurse in this situation. With the forthcoming clinical grades increase in pay in April and December, you can guess how we feel. Many of us have many valuable years of experience and some of us are as clinical as our grade I colleagues. Moreover, the PRB has done a lot of damage to the future of nursing. Grades G, H and I have become very highly paid while the non-nurses are questioning why they remain so poorly paid. Many of my grade I colleagues are very quiet about their pay because they never thought they would earn so much money.

As a result of these changes, many senior managers want the job to be done cheaper and, in the future, no clinical nurse would want to become a senior manager because of the poor pay. In ten to twenty years time the nurses' boss will be a senior manager who is not a nurse and doesn't understand many nursing issues. The only achievement of the PRB is, perhaps, to give junior grades better money, but the damage caused is immense.

Yours faithfully,

Patrick K S POON, RGN, CHSM, Assistant Nursing and Patients Services Manager, Burton General Hospital.

Status of Nursing Eroded

When I first came to Newmarket as a pupil nurse, my pay was £20 a month. The deductions included payment for accommodation and food and I thought it was good pay for a nineteen year old. However, for many years nurses' pay was regarded as very poor but, over the years, pay slowly improved. When I became a charge nurse in 1976 my pay wasn't too bad and five years later, when I became a nursing officer in charge of five ward sisters, I heard from one boastful sister that she was earning more than her sister and her husband put together.

The strenuous efforts made by hospital staff to draw attention to their heavy responsibilities and unbalanced pay structure put pressure on the government and led to the establishment of the Pay Awarding Body, and in 1991 the grading system was introduced. Suddenly, nurses' pay became very good and, because there were so many nurses working in the NHS, this became a major item of government expenditure. My letter rang true and several years later politicians and senior managers were looking for cheaper ways of providing nursing care in hospitals, or in an alternative care environment.

Care assistants, who were paid much less than nurses, were introduced and took over many roles previously performed by nurses. This eroded the status and role of nursing and there are now many non-nurse managers in charge of nursing staff, causing frustration and dissatisfaction on the wards. I am not saying that nurses didn't deserve better pay but, on the whole, the increases in pay have done the profession no favours.

The Pay Review Process of 1988.

The above letter, "PRB Fails Senior Managers" was written after the pay review.

When it was introduced in 1988, many nurses were placed on lower grades than the published criteria seemed to indicate. As a result, we set up a pay review meeting between those nurses who wished to contest their grading and senior management. I was a senior nurse who, together with a union representative, supported the case for the nurses against decisions made by some senior managers from another section.

It was a painful experience to see individual nurses putting a case to the panel and fighting for the grade and payment to which they claimed they were entitled. Some were winners and others were losers. I was in the middle, trying to represent and support nurses from different specialties, their claims being based on a variety of situations and roles. I often felt that a middle manager's job was a frustrating one, nowhere more so than during the long and painful Pay Review Process, and union officials felt the same.

As the years have gone by, nurses' pay has increased considerably, and because of the large numbers involved the increase has meant a substantial outlay of taxpayers' money. Although salary is only one factor in assessing the value of a person's career, I feel, on the whole, that most nurses ended up with a bad deal.

1988/1991

Tale 29
Hospitals v Nursing Homes

'*You pay your money and you takes your choice.*' Punch 1846

Working in NHS hospitals for twenty-seven years has given me a satisfactory and sheltered life. I was paid reasonably well and the terms and conditions of employment were very good, with generous sickness benefits and long holidays. The management structure was hierarchical and the culture bureaucratic. There were more and more forms to fill in, but slowly technology was coming into the hospitals.

When I left the NHS in 1996, I was fortunate that it didn't take me long to find a job as a trained nurse in a nursing home, starting as a staff nurse. It was a big climb-down for me to help bathing a patient again as I hadn't done that for years. The job was very different from what I had been used to, but I soon got used to it and learnt much from working in a totally different environment. The nurses at the homes were not paid very well at all, the terms and conditions were poor, holidays were shorter and there were no provisions for sick pay in many homes. Making money was a first priority, whereas there was so much waste and inefficiency in the NHS.

Why then did nurses work in nursing homes? Some were quite out of touch with the technological advances made in hospitals but many liked the much greater responsibility and accountability involved. The matron or manager of a care home had to go shopping for food for residents whereas hospital managers just rang the internal catering department to order whatever food was required. When a light bulb needed changing in a hospital, the nurse on the ward had to write out a requisition to the works department and it was not unusual to wait two weeks for it to be replaced. In a care home it was done by the handyman on the same day or, at most, the day after. I used to complain to the works department about this because it was often found that the requisition form was never received and when this happened it could take three weeks to have the bulb replaced. In my nursing home, the resident nun used to climb a ladder and change the bulb herself and I used to tease her by saying that it wasn't in her job description. In the NHS all staff had to adhere rigidly to their roles and one would never find a nurse changing a light bulb. There was no flexibility in the NHS, but many nurse matrons in care homes told me that they enjoyed the varied roles in the home, in spite of the fact that they weren't paid as well and had fewer holidays.

Nurses had many responsibilities in the homes. They didn't have house doctors nearby to call. They alone had to decide whether they should call a GP and decisions were much more individual than in hospitals, where second opinions were always readily available. The relationship between doctors and the residents and staff of care homes were more familiar and that was good for the residents. I once was asked by a GP if we should stop antibiotic treatment for an old lady who was suffering from her third stroke. She was dying from the third episode of a chest infection and her daughter had asked the GP to stop treating her mother. I simply said to him, "who am I to decide to withdraw a resident's treatment when I know it would end her life?"

He did decide to stop treating the old lady and she died soon afterwards. I was sure that his decision was correct as the lady did tell me when she was alive that she would rather die than suffer from any more chest infections, which made her feel so ill.

Quite often, the nurse in charge was the sole trained nurse on duty at the home and when the nurse in charge was unable to work because of illness there would be a panic, as finding another nurse always proved to be very difficult. Unlike hospitals, where there was a large pool of nurses, it was very difficult to find help for a care home at short notice, even from nursing agencies. It was not unusual to be working in a nursing home for longer than the twelve-hour shift because the trained nurse could not find a replacement to hand over to. According to the UK code of practice there should always be a trained nurse on duty in a nursing home, so trained nurses had no choice. The reality was that a trained nurse who had been working in excess of twelve hours would be much more likely to make a mistake and then who would take the blame?

I once did a survey of my students who were managers to find out why they continued to work in nursing homes. The main reason they gave was job satisfaction, followed by pay. Many managers felt unhappy in the NHS because of the bureaucracy and red tape. They felt tied to their jobs because of the good pay and terms and conditions, but it was a sorry state of affairs. However, those who worked in nursing homes had fewer employment rights. They were not represented by trade unions and coercion was common, whereas in the NHS union power was very evident.

There was much meanness and penny-pinching by the owners of care homes, such as diluting milk with water to reduce costs. The owner might limit how many incontinence pads residents were allowed to use and how many potatoes they were allowed to eat.

There were, however, many good nursing homes. My last nursing home was the first in which I saw good pastoral care in action. Resident nuns talked to patients frequently, with kindness and sincerity, encouraging them to unburden their minds by talking to someone they knew genuinely cared. The service was, of course, free. The nuns lived at the home with the residents and cared for them for as long as it was necessary. It was a privilege to see such wonderful care being practiced in the home.

1999

Tale 30
Project 2000

'Have no fear of perfection – you'll never reach it.'
Salvador Dali

Any nurse in the 1990s and 2000s would have heard of the term, "Project 2000." Project 2000 was a new programme of student nurse training and nurses had no choice but to embrace the new plan. It was designed by some academic nursing "thinktank" and was supposed to enhance nurse training and consequently improve nursing practice. All new entrants were required to have a degree, the training plan was different, and the emphasis seemed to be less on clinical experience and more on theoretical knowledge. Universities and classrooms seemed to be rated more highly than hospital wards.

At the same time there was to be only one grade of trained nurse, the registered general nurse. The clinical grade of state enrolled nurse was to disappear and all enrolled nurses had to cease working and be converted to registered general nurses.

Following this new concept of training and re-grading, who would do the clinical work? The new programme of nurse training wouldn't allow much time for clinical placements. The academics considered nurses were becoming expensive and, to save money, another grade should be introduced to do the clinical work such as bathing patients, making beds and emptying commodes, which were tasks nurses did under the old system. Care assistants, trained to a higher standard than the old grade of auxiliary nurse, were introduced to the wards nurses.

All these changes had a tremendous impact on the future of nursing. Firstly, Project 2000 student nurses were trained to become "desk nurses." Their clinical experience was less than half that required of the old training scheme. Once qualified, they were very good at paperwork and computers but they were unsure about helping with practical procedures such as helping doctors set up a trolley for an intravenous infusion, or for a lumbar puncture, and they certainly had to learn how to make a bed.

During Project 2000 training, students had only a few weeks of clinical placement to observe procedures and because of that they lacked practical experience. In fact, it was common knowledge that their presence was not regarded as a "pair of hands" to help out on the wards. Many nurses, like myself, from the old training system voiced our concerns but we were overruled. The project idea was imposed by the government and it would go ahead regardless. As a result, many newly qualified trained nurses from project 2000 were not recognised in their first year as a trained staff because their clinical performance on the ward was so poor. Only from their second year, would they be counted as staff nurses. What a waste of manpower and money!

It was no surprise that ten years later this system of training for nurses was reviewed and considered to be a failure. It was a good example of a training programme designed by academics for an essentially practical job. Meanwhile, the NVQ training of care assistants was progressing by leaps and bounds and soon they were trained to do many tasks previously done by nurses, such as taking blood, making beds, and removing secretions by tracheotomies in some specialties. In fact, other than giving out drugs, that only a trained nurse could do, the care assistants could fulfil most of the basic roles of a trained nurse. The care assistants were paid much less than staff nurses and wards were staffed with more care assistants and fewer trained nurses.

The irony was that NVQ trained care assistants had become the old state enrolled nurses, a clinical grade that had disappeared some fifteen years previously. What a circular game nursing had become!

In the 1990s I was one of the qualified nurses who objected to project 2000 and to NVQ training, the allegedly cheaper way of training clinical nurses, yet, fifteen years later I became an NVQ assessor and teacher. In a way, I had become a traitor but I lamented what the training of nurses had become. It had become an academic, knowledge based kind of training, rather than the development of the skills and attitudes required for the care of patients. There was no more throwing-in at the deep end on the wards, to learn as we worked, as in our good old days.

It is also true to say that NVQs have developed considerably over the years. We now have NVQ progression to level two, three, four and five, something no one thought possible in the 1990s. The National Vocational Qualification system has affected training at all levels throughout industry, not just in nursing, but in most service and productive industries, including accountancy, management and engineering.

2012

Tale 31
How Nursing Changed Me

'You cannot change what you refuse to confront.'
Everyday Life Lessons.

I have been a trained male nurse for thirty eight years. I came from Hong Kong to England in April 1969 and the first time I returned to Hong Kong was some five years later. Since then I have been very fortunate to go home every two or three years. I am very lucky to have a group of old college friends in Hong Kong and on every visit most of them turn up to meet me in a restaurant. We have dinner together and talk about old times and the changes that have occurred since my last visit.

Our friendship goes back some forty-five years and we have seen each other grow old and grey. In Hong Kong most people have to retire at sixty and therefore many of my friends are now retired. My frequent visits to Hong Kong have strengthened our friendship and advances in technology now enable us to maintain contact by email or face book. It is a friendship we treasure.

Two years ago, at a restaurant, we met a lady we

nicknamed "Indian" because when she was younger, she would tie her hair in two bundles at the back, like an Indian. Nine of us were sitting around the table, enjoying the food and, more importantly, each other's company.

"Patrick," she asked, "do you remember when you were fifteen or sixteen, every time you stood up, your face blushed so much?"

"Yes, like a red faced soldier," I replied, "I remember it well. Who would have thought that now I can talk confidently to strangers and have some social skills? I have been teaching for ten years and have been standing in front of a group of managers and it doesn't bother me at all."

"I can see a big change in you," Indian said.

"Yes, nursing has changed me so much. Time and nursing have enabled me to greet new patients I have never met before. As a charge nurse, I met many people and, as a manager in the NHS, I have had some good training in teaching and presentation skills. Mind you, it has aged me quite a bit too."

"Well, you look good for your age."

"Yes, I have been lucky. Nursing and teaching are both rewarding jobs; seeing patients get better and students successfully completing their courses. I have seen nurses progressing into tutors, managers and senior professionals, and they have been thankful."

"Lucky you," one old friend said.

"That's why I am an advocate for nursing. It has given me a good life and I'm grateful."

"What is the down side then?" a friend asked.

"Well, I have worked very long days, some, in a nursing home, as long as twelve hours. It was unsafe really as I was very tired, and the responsibilities sometimes weighed heavily upon me. As a nursing officer, there were times when I went home after work worried." "Worried about what?" my friend asked.

"I was very worried that we didn't have enough staff to do the work, and most of the other wards were the same. We only had time to do the basic jobs."

"Well, the NHS in England is better than medical care here in Hong Kong!"

"Yes, I know that the nurses in Hong Kong work very hard and that they are busier than nurses in England."

I had a good dinner with my old friends. We had studied together at Tung Chi College in Wanchai, Hong Kong, for five years in the 1960s when we were in our teens. The old college has now been demolished. My friends became accountants, engineers and bank workers. We said our farewells and wished each other good luck. God bless you all, old friends.

The world of nursing changed me from a shy and immature youth into a confident, experienced man with social skills and I am very grateful for that.

2013

Tale 32
The saddest patient – 1997

'The living dead?'

I was working in a nursing home as a deputy matron/trainer. I was on an early shift from 7.30 in the morning. The time was 09.30 and most residents were helped and got up by the carers, eating their breakfast. I recalled the following conversation:

'Patrick, please go and have a word with Steve, would you? He is so difficult.' A care assistant informed me.

'Oh? What has he done?'

'He refused to get dress and has been rude and horrible to us and at present he is totally naked sitting on the toilet.'

'It's a cold morning.....'

'And he was f...ing and bl...ding this morning to all of us.'

I shook me head. I agreed and accepted tersely. 'I'll have a word with him.'

It was a late October morning and chill was in the air. Fortunately, the home was normally warm. I went upstairs to see Steve.

His room was cold as he wanted the windows open.

Steve was 70 years old, sane and mentally alert. He had been diagnosed with severe Parkinson's disease, he was constantly shaking (a type of palsy) that he needed constant care which could include direct care like feeding, dressing, washing and assisted ambulation. The sad fact was that mentally, he knew what was going on around him but could not physically control most if not all of his movements. The following dialogue unfolded.

'Morning, Steve.'

'Morning, Patrick.'

'What is the matter? Why did you not let the staff dress you for breakfast?'

'I don't feel like it.'

'You will miss breakfast.'

'I don't care.'

'OK, but please do not swear at the staff. They are not here to be sworn at.'

'But they won't leave me alone.'

'But they want to get the jobs done and get you dressed.'

'I don't care.'

'You will get cold then...'

'Mm.' Steve was a very stubborn man, ex-engineer and had lived in the home for 2 years. He was never married. Only a sister visited him at times.

'Shall I leave you to it then?'

He did not answer. We could not force him to dress nor to eat. There was no more I could do to help him.

I left the room for 30 minutes and the bell in his room rang. I was annoyed and went up to his room. I opened his door.

'Well, Steve.'

'I am cold.'

'Shall I ask someone to dress you?'

'OK.'

'Only if you let us do it for you 30 minutes ago.'

He did not answer.

Steve was dressed by the staff and missed his breakfast and he later had his lunch. He was fed and ate the lunch well.

Two months later, I applied and got a better job elsewhere. On my last day of the work in the nursing home, Steve was sitting near me and said, 'Patrick, with our differences, I wish you all the very best.'

'Thank you, Steve.'

There was a silence.

'Patrick, have you seen a Parkinson's sufferer so bad like me?'

'No, I am very sorry. I have not. And you have had it for 6 years now.'

'Yes, I wish I was dead. Mentally I am so sane and physically I cannot do anything, I cannot eat, poo, dress, nothing! I am a living dead! There is nothing worse than knowing that I cannot do what I used to do.'

I did not know what to say. My silence probably spoke volumes. Steve remained the saddest patient that I have seen. I have seen many patients dying, suffering from chronic diseases but all not for so long. And when they were poorly, they were delirious and did not know what was going on. I was mindful that many terminal patients were put on drugs to make them euphoric before they died. It was a much kinder way. Yet, here Steve was condemned to a death sentence with the date of execution indefinitely postponed.

In many nursing homes, one could see many 'living dead'

residents. Nora was another typical lady, paralysed by strokes and survived only by a tube feed into her stomach. She could not speak though she might know what was going on. We kept her alive by tube feeding her for two years. She was about 50 years old. It was the saddest thing to see a human being alive like that. If it was an animal like so, one would put it down as an act of kindness.

Unfortunately, there were many residents like Nora and Steve in the care homes up and down the country, totally dependent on carers to help them and most of them could not speak or appreciate any quality of life. I sometimes question the ethos of our care system. What do you think?

33

My old friend and me, the sea.

We meet again, my old friend , the sea.
Its blue waters and the azure sky, above me.

In my home town of Hong Kong, I am nearer to you, the sea.
Ferry across the harbour on your eternal smoothness, by me.

In the winters in Cornwall, I see the foam blown by,
from the sea, so cold and wild.

With thick coat and woolly hat on,
I roam on the beach, singing a winter song.

In the summer, I bodysurf on your waters,
Relishing the thrill it matters.

With exhilarating speed, you gave me a terrific ride to the shore,
On the swirling surf board, with the seagulls singing above, who could ask for more?

But in the summer, the time has gone too fast,
With your good company, it did not last.

But it is good to be by your side again, the sea.
The interminable horizon, the long beach and me.

You have been near me for the most of my life, you and me.
My old friend and me, the sea.

Patrick K S Poon.
December, 2012.

Tale 34
Looking Back – The Turning Points of My Career

'I am a slow walker but I never walk back.' Abraham Lincoln.

When I reflect upon my career in nursing I am aware that I reacted rashly in some situations, but fortunately the outcome in the long term was favourable. The main reason for my success in life was that I kept on studying, so my wife and part-time secretary told me.

When I first qualified in 1974, I was given the opportunity to be seconded to do a Diploma in Nursing and I took up the challenge with a few other qualified nurses. It was said to be a very difficult course but I studied hard and took the examinations. Out of ten students only a ward sister and I passed and I was thrilled and happy.

When a junior sister's post became available I applied, thinking that I was more qualified than the other applicants, and therefore I should get the post. However, the hospital appointed a staff nurse less experienced than I was. I was annoyed and walked out of the hospital. I was living in the nurses' home and I must have been naïve. If I resigned where would I live? Fortunately the Nursing Officer came to my home to compromise and I was offered a transfer back to casualty, which I loved. On reflection, now I am older and wiser, I should not have done this because I could have lost my job. When I was back in work in casualty, I continued to apply and was soon offered a promotion although it involved a change of location. I didn't mind as I was single and mobile.

After I left the hospital I kept in touch with the Charge Nurse in casualty and thirty years on, I found out from him that the sister's post wasn't given to me because I was Chinese and male. The hospital then preferred female nurses. It was obviously a discrimination issue, but the Sex Discrimination and Race Relations Acts of 1975 and 1976 had barely reached the statute book. To survive as a male nurse in the women-dominated world of nursing was not easy. But such was life then.

When I became a Charge Nurse and then a Nursing Officer in Walsall, I took the opportunity to take a course on data processing management. I knew that computerisation was coming in and needed to learn a different skill. We were very fortunate in the NHS and I was seconded to the course with time off and financial help.

From the 1980s, NHS had a reorganisation every three years. The management structure was changed regularly; roles were renamed and involved more responsibility for the same payment. People had different bosses nearly every time following a reorganisation. It was Hobson's choice.

In 1986 I applied for a new post in a new structure and didn't get it. Another newcomer who was English was given my job. He was my student nurse but he had an oily mouth and he moved on speedily. Fortunately, I had a senior nursing officer, Mrs. Hever, who enjoyed working with me and asked for my transfer to help her. It was a lucky escape and I was much happier in the post but I knew it was a temporary position and soon I applied elsewhere. Because I had passed the first year of the data processing management course, I was offered a better post than I had applied for in the new structure. I became a deputy director of Burton Hospitals and was in sole charge of a local general hospital. The hospital had ten wards, including medical and surgical wards, which I had good experience of. It wasn't a bad job for a 37 year old man.

One lesson I had learnt was that one had to keep on training and learning to survive and to keep a job. If you stayed still, you would be overtaken. As one got older, it would also become more difficult to find a good job. I always admired what Abraham Lincoln said, "I am a slow walker but I never walk back."

You might have heard of a Chinese folk tale which goes like this:

On a farm, there was a man and his son Hui raising horses for a living. They were neither rich nor poor but could make a living, using the horses to help to plough the field and grow crops. They were happy, but one day thunder and lightning came, the worst they had seen for a long time, and the horses escaped. Hui and his father cried, and said, "It is going to be very hard to make a living now."

Two days later, war was declared and the government went to the villages to recruit men to fight. All the young men with horses had to go to war and no man would have a choice. They went to Hui's village and took all the men with horses to war but Hui wasn't taken because he didn't have a horse. The moral of the tale was that losing something might be good for you in the long run.

The pattern of my nursing career seemed to repeat itself. I was a reader of The Nursing Times, a professional nursing journal and I wrote an article which was published in December 2004. This is that article:

"Change can be a good thing."

Sometimes, when you reflect on events, good or bad, you can be grateful for what happened. You might not have felt so at the time, but later on you count it as a blessing.

This is how I feel when I look back at the events that led me to leave the NHS and start a career working in nursing homes.

I had worked as an operational manager and nursing officer for surgical units in two NHS hospitals for fourteen years. I reached the point where I felt I had seen all there was to see and there was no longer a challenge or excitement. I didn't know what I wanted to do.

In 1996, when there was yet another reorganisation, I was offered another post with protected pay and wasn't happy. Fortunately, with help and good advice, I got a very good deal from the NHS, in addition to my pension.

When I left the NHS, I had been in nursing for twenty-seven years and had been through the ranks of staff nurse, charge nurse and nursing officer. Having been promoted young, I guess I was suffering from 'burnout'. I had never worked outside the NHS and I was feeling nervous about the future. Fortunately, I soon got a job in a nursing home and soon became a deputy matron in another home nearby. Since then, I have worked in another two nursing homes as a deputy matron and trainer and gained valuable experience in care management.

I had always enjoyed teaching students and qualified nurses in the NHS, so I decided to take on a role of a NVQ trainer for carers. I studied and gained the relevant qualifications and then became a part time lecturer at a local college. I subsequently secured a full-time post teaching outreach NVQs and care management and from 2003, I started teaching the Registered Managers' Award. Every year, I taught something different and enjoyed the change.

My final year in the NHS was stressful. I feared leaving, but doing so proved to be the turning point of my career. I now work not so much for money, but for satisfaction and enjoyment, so if you are going through another change or reorganisation and your position is in danger, don't despair. It may be a blessing in disguise. If I knew what I know now, I would not have been so worried.

Patrick Poon, RGN, DHSM, Cert.Ed, lecturer at Stephenson College, Leicestershire.

The article was read by a colleague at my college who enjoyed reading it and when I went into the town, I met a woman who once worked for me on the surgical unit. It made my day when she told me she had read my article and relished the experience.

Some two years later, at the College where I worked, I received a letter from a nurse who had read my article in the Nursing Times and kept it. She commented how it had inspired her and encouraged her in her work. I was so touched that I replied and wished her luck. The article was written in 2012, and some eight years later I am fortunate to still be employed and doing interesting work. I have now been working for an awarding body as an accreditation officer, standard verifier and moderator. In addition, I also enjoy working with NVQs students at a local college.

I have indeed good cause to count my blessings.

2013